BONE BOOSTERS

NATURAL WAYS TO BEAT OSTEOPOROSIS

BOXTREE

DIANA MORAN
AND
HELEN FRANKS

The authors wish to thank the following:

Carol Jones, Osteoporosis Prevention Officer, Dorset HealthCare Trust Headquarters, Shelley Road, Bournemouth, Dorset.

Dr Paul Thompson, MD, MRCP, Consultant Rheumatologist, Poole Hospital Trust, Poole, Dorset.

Linda Whike, MCSP, SRP, Grad. Dip Phys., BWT Chartered Physiotherapists, 41 Church Road, Parkstone, Poole, Dorset.

Emma Robshaw and Lorraine Scott, Department of Nutrition and Dietetics, Royal Bournemouth and Christchurch Hospitals Trust, Dorset.

Everett Smith, Department of Preventative Medicine, University of Wisconsin for research papers on ageing, exercise and osteoporosis.

First published in Great Britain in 1993

This updated edition published in 1995 by Boxtree Limited, Broadwall House, 21 Broadwall, London SE1 9PL.

Illustrations by Greg Mason.
Designed and typeset by Blackjacks, London.
Printed and bound in Finland by WSOY

A CIP catalogue entry for this book is available from the British Library.

ISBN 1 85283 933 3

Front cover photograph courtesy of Graeme Ainscough.

CONTENTS

BONE BOOSTERS:

The total lifeplan to strengthen bones

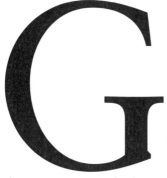REEN GODDESS exercise specialist Diana Moran and medical writer Helen Franks first got together when working on a feature about fitness for women in mid-life. Within minutes they were talking about the importance of keeping bones strong at the menopause and what scientists were discovering about the way exercise could help guard against osteoporosis, the bone-thinning condition that affects one woman in four after the menopause. HRT, they agreed, though extremely helpful for very many women, was not the complete answer. Exercise to strengthen bones and make for all-round fitness and flexibility was essential. If this was true for women taking HRT, it was even more important for those who chose not to, either because they had a medical history that made the treatment unsuitable, or because they preferred not to take hormones on a long-term basis, or because they found that HRT just did not suit them. Out of their conversations, and their determination to stay fit themselves, came the idea for *Bone Boosters*.

Why we wrote this book

Diana: 'I have been interested in all forms of movement and sport since I was a little girl. I enjoy being active in my work and my play and have taught exercise for over 25 years.

It all started informally when I was in my late 20s. My girlfriends commented on my zest for life and my posture, and asked for advice on how to keep fit. I taught them what I knew about a healthy diet, and showed them my exercise techniques, many of which I had used in my former athletics training, plus exercises I had been given by hospital physiotherapists during and after my pregnancies. I was always on the look-out for new, safe and effective exercises.

Gradually, the whole thing snowballed and I went on to teach holiday-makers for many years in West Country holiday camps. My TV début as an exercise teacher occurred in the late 1970s and hailed the birth of the Green Goddess.

During the 1980s when I was with BBC Breakfast Time, fitness became fashionable, but injuries were reported by some doctors and physiotherapists as the result of intensive high-impact aerobics. Exercise teachers became concerned, and some of us got together to form ASSET (the Association of Exercise Teachers, now known as The Exercise Association of England). We decided standards needed to be set and the gaining of qualifications encouraged, and many of us conscientiously went back to school to learn more. I and many others gained the necessary qualifications for the teaching of safe and effective exercise to music, and I went on to gain specialist skills in the teaching of the 50-plus adult, with whom I personally feel a great affinity, being in that age group myself.

I suppose being 50-plus, I should have thought twice about leading a party of similarly-aged friends on an ice-skating jaunt to a newly-opened ice rink in Poole, Dorset, in 1990. "Pride comes before a fall" was the painful lesson I was to learn. I slipped and – crack! – it was all so easy.

A Colles fracture (broken wrist) was diagnosed, and I received first-hand experience of just how painful and inconvenient breaking bones can be. I was only to regain full use of my wrist – vital for my work – through extensive physio-therapy and a great deal of discomfort. The experience focused my attention on osteoporosis, particularly as the break I had received was one common among sufferers from that condition. The disease osteoporosis had interested me for several years: so much so, in fact, that after reading an article about it in the *Daily Mail* in 1988, I had taken myself off to the Amarant Clinic in London to investigate. I was interested in claims that HRT could help prevent the thinning of bones. Green Goddesses need strong bones!

I was 48 at the time, and pre-menopausal. The clinic doctor insisted upon an obligatory "mid-life service", as I called it, before making any decisions or giving any opinions as to my suitability for Hormone Replacement Therapy. I

Exercise before and after the menopause offers similar protection against bone loss. Evidence comes from a 4-year follow-up of 8 women aged between 35 and 65, some pre- and others post-menopausal. They went on a 3-day-a-week exercise routine consisting of 10 minutes warm-up, 30 minutes aerobic activity (including dancing and jogging), and 5 minutes cool-down. Arm-bone thickness was compared over the years with a matched group who did no exercise. At the start, the exercise group was found to be less fit than the control group, but gradually they switched. The rate of bone loss was different too, with a significant reduction in loss in the areas measured. The researchers predicted that only 5% of bone would be lost in the exercisers over 20 years, compared to 25% in the non-exercisers.

entered the clinic feeling fit and fine, but on leaving I found I had an unexpected problem. A mammogram, part of the MOT, had revealed irregularities, and breast cancer was diagnosed. However, it was in its early stages and therefore could be treated successfully. Two months after surgery I resumed some of my work, although it took several more months to regain the necessary strength and stamina required to perform and teach exercise.

Medical opinion is divided over whether women with a history of breast cancer like myself should take HRT, either to relieve the symptoms of the menopause or to lessen the risk of thinning bones. I decided I must find out more. Some months later I met author and medical journalist Helen Franks while working on a project concerned with fitness, and we quickly came to the same conclusion. There was a need to investigate developments in the treatment of osteoporosis and to devise a bone-strengthening exercise plan based on the latest research.'

Helen: 'One of the first health features I ever wrote for a women's magazine was on the subject of HRT. That was back in the 1970s when the medical profession paid little

---

A hysterectomy or womb removal brings on an early menopause with the resultant upheaval in hormone balance. This means a woman in perhaps her early 30s is in danger of experiencing bone thinning and needs medical advice on how to combat it. Even when the ovaries are not removed, they cease to function in the majority of women within 2 to 4 years after hysterectomy.

> *Poor posture carries its own risk of broken bones. Recent research suggests that an unstable walk with body sway is associated with hip fractures. The underlying cause is thought to be poor muscle tone, especially in the legs. So Bone Boosters, which also, of course, boost the muscles, reduce the risk factor in two ways.*

regard to menopausal symptoms and most doctors had barely heard of this condition of thinning bones called osteoporosis. I wrote up news from America about HRT, an effective treatment against short and long-term effects of the menopause.

Then came the finding that HRT could cause cancer of the womb lining – endometrial cancer – and the treatment was altered to combine oestrogen with progestogen, so that women would experience monthly "breakthrough bleeding" which meant a regular shedding of the womb lining. Only those who had a hysterectomy would now receive "unopposed oestrogen".

At this time I was a health editor of a women's magazine, and I began to receive letters from readers worrying about the new findings, wanting to keep strong bones but concerned about the possible hazards of taking a drug regularly for many years. Even with the assurance that the combined HRT treatment was safe, there were women who felt it was not for them. Some had breast cancer, others had a history of non-malignant lumps and cysts and were worried about taking a hormone treatment when there was no long-term research into risks and side effects. Then there were the ones who gave up after 6 months or so because they suffered fluid retention, weight gain or breast tenderness when on HRT, or who

> *A short course of steroids is unlikely to have a bad effect on bones. It's the continual need for steroids that can be a problem, for instance when they are taken regularly as a treatment for arthritis or to prevent asthma. There's no way of predicting who will or will not lose bone through taking steroids regularly. Exercise, especially the regime shown in* Bone Boosters, *and a calcium-rich diet, will offer protection.*

found the return of periods unacceptable. And the ones who had been told that their medical condition precluded them from the treatment. What were they to do?

By the time I joined the 50-plus age group I could understand all too well their concerns. There are still no long-term, large-scale research findings on HRT. Women still experience unwelcome side effects, and that basic dislike of being on a course of drugs for a long time is still prevalent. I also realised that taking the hormone treatment was no antidote to the odd aches and pains and stiffness of growing older. Exercise was essential, and if HRT was off the agenda, then exercise designed specifically to strengthen bones was top priority.

I'm lucky enough to live near Hampstead Heath, so I walk there regularly, winter and summer, come drizzle or shine. I go to a yoga class twice a week, and tap dancing once a week. All very good for bones, of course, but a bit hit and miss. I knew of the mounting body of research regarding bone-strengthening exercise, and then I met Diana. The result is *Bone Boosters*.'

Do you want what we want?

What we wanted was a simple set of exercises that we could fit into our daily lives with the minimum of fuss. These should be scientifically designed to put stress on bones and thus increase strength – especially important in the years coming up to the menopause and immediately after, though useful for women of all ages.

We also wanted a complete update on everything we needed to know about keeping ourselves fit and healthy so that we could enjoy life into ripe old age. So we added information on diet and alternative nutrition to help make healthy bones, plus the latest developments in drug and hormone treatments, the sports and leisure activities that give our bones a 'boost', and all the medical findings on osteoporosis to put us completely in the picture. We've also included a special Osteo-Relief section for women who already suffer from osteoporosis, with tailor-made exercises to help ease the condition and stop it from progressing.

Do you want what we want?

If you do, it's all here in *Bone Boosters*.

Hibernating bears may provide a clue to bone loss. Despite months of inactivity when hibernating, they manage to recycle bone and wake up in springtime with strong skeletons. Researchers hope one day to identify the chemical that works the miracle and apply it to humans.

WHAT IS OSTEOPOROSIS?

E'VE BEEN hearing a great deal about this bone-thinning condition in recent times, but it is by no means new. The Romans were referring to non-healing hip fractures and other similar-sounding conditions in the 6th century. By the early 19th century, physicians were concerned about the 'spongy' texture of bones in old age, even before they were able to see them on X-ray.

Today, we regard osteoporosis as a preventable disease, though there is still a great deal we don't know about it. Despite its association with ageing and the menopause, the condition can also affect younger women and men. Though more cases are being diagnosed, it doesn't necessarily follow that incidences are rising. There are also the facts that more of us are living longer, and that doctors are more aware of the effects of bone-thinning. But other reasons for more cases

---

Two common causes of missing and irregular periods in younger women can lead to bone loss. One is anorexia. A study of young women suffering from anorexia and missing periods for a year showed that 77% had spinal bone loss. Poor nutrition, weight loss and loss of ovarian function were the causes. Though exercise in normal amounts is protective, too much of it is definitely a bad thing. When young women athletes train to excess, they become underweight, their periods stop, and they can lose 5% of bone density a year.

of osteoporosis could be excessive dieting, poor nutrition, or lack of exercise and sedentary lifestyles.

It is estimated that 1 in 4 women will suffer from a fracture in later life because of loss of bone density.

What are bones made of?

Bone consists of the compound calcium phosphate embedded in collagen fibres. The calcium gives strength and hardness, the fibres make for flexibility. There are two types of bone: trabecular and cortical. A woman will lose about 50% of trabecular bone and 35% of cortical bone in her lifetime. Trabecular bone is most likely to be lost in the 10 years or so around the menopause. Cortical bone is associated with slower, gradual bone loss later in life.

The forearms and spinal column are made up largely of trabecular bone, and fractures in these areas are a sign of post-menopausal osteoporosis. Hip and shoulder bones are both cortical and trabecular. Fractures here are associated with later ageing.

> *Taking the pill may protect against bone loss. There's some evidence that women who have taken oral contraceptives for a long time have denser bones than women who have not. The hormones in oral contraceptives may stimulate release of a substance called calcitonin which inhibits bone breakdown.*

Bone tissue is continually replacing itself, most rapidly in the young and more moderately in adulthood. Peak bone mass is reached during the early 20s, and after that, if you want to look at it pessimistically, things begin to go downhill. In women, bone loss at around the age of 30 is up to 1% a year. In men, the rate is slower until middle age. This gradual loss of bone density is common to everyone and is part of the ageing process. But in some women, the loss accelerates to between 2% and 3% a year at the onset of the menopause, and by the age of 70, a third of bone mineral mass can have disappeared. You can see the results in the skinny ankles and so-called 'dowager's hump' or stoop of some elderly women. That stoop is the result of what are known as crush fractures in the spine.

What happens at the menopause?

A natural drop in levels of the hormone oestrogen at the menopause triggers an accelerated loss of calcium from the bone. One of the mysteries surrounding osteoporosis is that though all women lose oestrogen at the menopause, not all of them suffer bone loss. There are certain risk factors that make some women more vulnerable than others – more about this below. The increased loss occurs at whatever age the menopause takes place, whether it's at 35 or 50, whether it comes on naturally or through removal of the womb and ovaries for medical reasons.

The risk factors

- Heavy drinking and smoking
- Heavy caffeine intake
- Slight build, low weight
- Menopause before the age of 45
- Family history of osteoporosis, especially in close female relatives, i.e. mother or grandmother
- Lack of exercise
- Prolonged bed rest or immobility
- Fair skin
- Lack of sufficient calcium in diet throughout life
- High protein diet – increases calcium loss
- Vitamin D deficiency – reduces body's ability to utilise calcium
- Long course of cortisone or thyroid treatment
- Anorexia

Your weight at the age of 1 year could predict bone strength in adult life. A study of 230 women whose weight at 1 year was traced from old records showed that those who were under-average in weight in infancy did not develop as strong a skeleton in adulthood as bigger babies. Results were the same in two different age groups – women now aged 21 as well as those aged 68.

What are the effects of bone loss?

There may be nothing noticeable at first. It's what happens in the long run that counts. A typical sign is the broken wrist (Colles fracture). You know the scenario: the person slips and falls on an outstretched hand. Her average age will be 60 – and we use the word 'she' advisedly because it happens much more often to women than to men.

Fracture of the femur, the thigh bone, is another indicator. It can happen through quite a minor fall. The incidence rises with increased age in both men and women, but again it's women who are statistically more prone to these injuries.

And then there are fractures of the vertebrae, or spine. They become more frequent from the age of 50, again primarily in women. They can cause loss of height through a concave or wedging effect of the weakened bones, or the spinal column may collapse because the bones are actually crushed. One estimate suggests that about 60% of elderly women will experience wedging of bones in the spine.

Hip fractures increase after the age of 70, and are the most serious of the four types of fracture connected with osteoporosis. While the other kinds may cause pain, they rarely need much medical care. But hip fractures are associated with hospitalisation, permanent disability and death in old age.

In the 1960s there were around 10,000 hip fractures a year in the UK. By the 1990s we're talking in terms of nearer 40,000. Never mind the financial burden – some £500 million a year to the NHS – there's also the cost in human misery and pain. Yet we say again – some osteoporosis is preventable.

> *Heavier women gain extra protection in two ways. Greater body weight puts more stress on the bones (just as exercise does). And, after the menopause, where's there's fat there's also the chance to store more oestrogen – in the fat cells.*

All fall down

Fractures follow falls. Even a minor impact can lead to a fracture when bones reach a certain stage of brittleness. Why do people fall down more as they get older?

There are a number of reasons. They could be on a course of drug treatment that makes them drowsy or lose balance – tranquillisers, for instance. They may suffer from muscular weakness through illness or lack of exercise. Vision may not be as keen so there's the danger of tripping over, especially where lighting is not too good either, for instance in a hall or on stairs. Blackouts or fainting due to a physical condition are further hazards. Cold weather too can take its toll. One study of elderly women admitted to hospital with fractures showed that there was a mid-winter peak. But they weren't slipping on icy pavements; most of the accidents took place indoors. The researchers noted that a large proportion of the women were thin, possibly suffering from poor nutrition which can trigger low body temperature, hypothermia and subsequent lack of coordination.

The value of screening

The good news is that it's possible to measure bone loss, the best time to do it being around the menopause. The bad news is that this is no reliable way of predicting who will later suffer fractures. Only about a third of women found to have low bone density through screening are likely to experience fractures in later life.

Screening is useful, however, as a predictor and a way of signalling the need for a healthier lifestyle. Ideally, it should be offered to any woman under 70 with thin bones, or who is known to be at risk of oestrogen deficiency, or who has been on steroids long-term. Various techniques for screening are now being offered to women over 50, in some NHS hospitals and also at private menopause clinics, though at present there are no plans for nationwide screening.

Screening techniques

'Screening for osteoporosis is like measuring the shadow of a tree,' says consultant radiologist Dr Jim Stevenson. In other words, an inexact process. Most ways of measuring that

> *Women who smoke experience menopause on average three years earlier than non-smokers. And if you live with a smoker, but don't smoke yourself, you're at the same disadvantage. The earlier the menopause, the earlier the risk of thinning bones.*

shadow involve the use of machines known as 'densitometers'. These expose bones to small doses of radiation, considered to be well within safety limits. One method, with the cumbersome name of Single Photon Absorptiometry, measures the bone density of the wrist. You rest your wrist under the machine, with a cuff wrapped round the forearm, and results are conveniently displayed on screen within five minutes. Dual Photo Absorptiometry (usually known as DEXA) is a more advanced screening method, being faster, more accurate and able to measure bone density of the spinal column, thigh bones and also other bones if necessary.

There is some debate over where best to measure to get accurate results. A side view of the spine is thought to be most suitable for people over the age of 70, but this involves a higher radiation dose than, say, a scan of the thigh bone. One problem with current versions of scanning is that there is no simple relationship between the state of bones in different parts of the body. You could be losing bone in the wrist but not in the hip, for instance.

There are various versions of DEXA, all involving lying on a couch before the results are shown on a computer screen. Latest models will read out in 2–10 minutes, depending on body area. As a rough guide, the quicker the

Studies in the United States show that black people have stronger, thicker, larger bones than the white population. Black women tend to lose bone more slowly than white women; and they lose less calcium in their urine than white women. Black and white men, on the other hand, lose bone and calcium in similar amounts.

read-out, the more modern the machine and the lower the dose of radiation.

A new alternative to body scanners is the Achilles Ultrasound bone densitometer, which, as its name suggests, uses ultrasound not radiation and scans the heel. This area is pure trabecular bone and is considered to be a good indicator of body bone loss, though again there's some doubt about whether the state of the heel bone is a true guide to, for instance, the state of the thigh bone. With this method, the foot is immersed in heated water and the reading comes up on the computer screen in 5 minutes in graph form, showing whether bone thickness is above or below average for age.

HOW OUR EXERCISE PROGRAMME CAN HELP YOU

Our *BONE BOOSTERS* PROGRAMME consists of a set of easy movements designed specifically to strengthen and preserve bone thickness. They are exercises you can do in your everyday life, around your home or workplace or in the garden. You need no more than 20–30 minutes a day, for three days a week, though we do ask that you build up to this slowly to avoid possible injury or over-tiring.

Bone Boosters are intended especially for women of 40-plus who are approaching the menopause, but the earlier you start incorporating them into your life, the better. There is also a special Osteo-Relief section of exercises for those who already suffer from osteoporosis.

But before you start this or any exercise programme, please check with your doctor if you suffer from heart disease, have high blood-pressure, joint problems, back problems, if you are very overweight, have any serious illness, or are convalescing.

If you already have osteoporosis, do not attempt the main Bone Boosters section and before starting on the special Osteo-Relief section, check with your doctor.

Before performing any of the exercises in your home or even out in the garden, it is essential that you check the supports and equipment you'll be using to make sure they are strong enough to take your weight.

To be effective, exercise must be done on a *regular* basis – some physical activity should be undertaken for an hour at least once a week, but preferably, less and more often. What is ideally required is a generally more active lifestyle. All exercise is good for us – inactivity isn't.

We know that it's a natural process for women and men to lose some density from bone after the age of 35. Research over the past 10 years or so has shown that through regular, weight-bearing exercise it is possible to prevent some of the dramatic loss often occuring in women over 50, largely due to the fall in levels of the female hormone oestrogen at the time of the menopause or earlier if there has been a premature menopause brought about by hysterectomy. Genetic inheritance and other factors can also contribute to bone loss.

Weight-bearing exercises or movements which use the body's own weight help preserve or even build bone. The effect only occurs when the weight is repeatedly exerted. Muscles attached to either end of a bone force it to twist and bend in response to the strike action and jarring movements. This stress-strengthening effect on the bone is boosted if sufficient calcium and Vitamin D are available – more on this in our chapter on nutrition.

Simple brisk walking, skipping or running use a hard, vibrating strike action, with the weight of the upper body borne by the spine, hips, legs and feet. A push-up uses whole body weight to strengthen shoulders, arms and wrists. Recent studies by Dr Joan Bassey at the Queen's Medical Centre, Nottingham, have shown that pre-menopausal women who were encouraged to do a series of little jumps for a controlled period of time, on a regular basis, significantly increased the bone density of their ankles, knees and femeral head.

Specific bones can be targeted still further by introducing additional weights. For example, exercising with dumb-bells puts extra demand on the arms and wrists. So does carrying heavy bags of shopping (so long as you keep a straight back and don't stoop). Lifting household objects, like heavy cooking pots or the vacuum cleaner, has a similar Bone-

Boosting effect. Twisting off a tight lid on a jar helps wrists and forearms too. Once you've followed our exercises, you'll be able to adapt other everyday objects and activities and turn them into your own Bone Boosters.

Our *Bone Boosters* programme targets hips, wrists, and spine in particular, these being the most vulnerable to the painful, crippling and sometimes fatal fractures caused as a result of osteoporosis. So go ahead, enjoy the sessions. Make them a part of your life – and may the power they bring be with you.

BONE BOOSTERS EXERCISE PLAN

B EFORE WE BEGIN our special Bone Boosters exercises, it is essential to warm-up by putting our major joints through their natural range of movement. This helps maintain mobility, warms up major muscles and raises the pulse. By adding some stretches, we will then be ready to continue exercising without the risk of injury. But the less fit you are, the longer you need to warm-up. An average warm-up will take 5–10 minutes.

WARM-UP

So, let's make a start. You need to be wearing loose, comfortable clothes and sports shoes if possible. Clear enough space and use furniture and fittings around the house, like tables, chairs, banisters and the kitchen sink, for support. Or better still, you could exercise outside in the fresh air. But before performing any exercises in your home or garden, it is essential to check that the support is secure and strong enough to take your weight, and that the ground surface you are working on isn't wet or slippery. Don't exercise until at least an hour after meals, and keep drinking water near at hand to avoid becoming dehydrated.

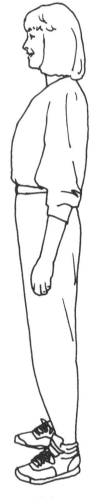

1 Stand Tall

Check your posture by standing with your feet comfortably apart, your shoulders back but down and relaxed. (Don't poke your head forward.) Pull in your tummy muscles, tighten your bottom and tuck your tail under. This will tilt your pelvis forward. Your knees should be soft (relaxed).

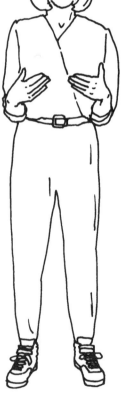

2 Wrist Circles

To mobilise wrists, sit in your chair or stand up. Tuck your elbows into your waist or place them on a table for support and simply circle your hands, working the wrists first 8 times in one direction, then 8 times in the other direction.

3 Windmills

To mobilise shoulders and release tension, place your finger-tips on your shoulders. Bring your elbows together in front of you, then take them up, and back, and draw imaginary circles with your elbows, pulling your shoulder blades apart – 8 times clockwise, then 8 times anti-clockwise.

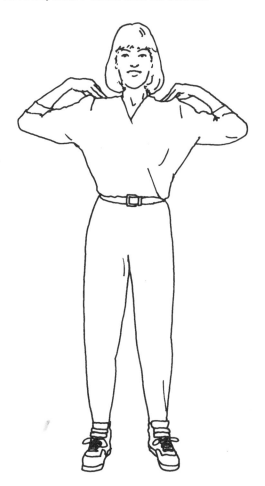

4 Head Rolls

To mobilise neck and release tension, look over your right shoulder with chin parallel to floor. Slowly drop your chin to your chest and roll it on to look over your left shoulder. Return your chin to your chest and back up to the right side. Continue, with control, 8 times. **Do not roll your head backwards.**

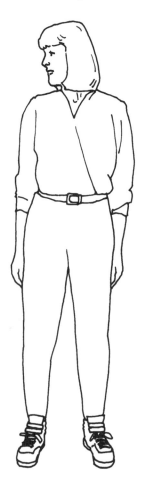

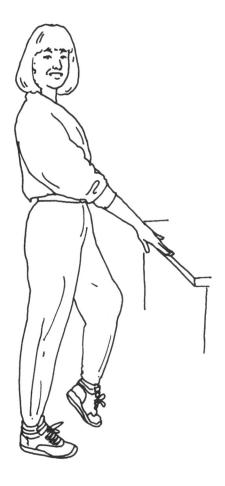

5 Ankle Circles

To mobilise ankles and toes, stand with your feet comfortably apart, hands on your hips or hold on to a table unit or
chair back for support. Place the toes of your right foot on
the ground. Keep them in place, heel up. Circle your ankle 8
times clockwise, then 8 times anti-clockwise. Repeat with
your left foot.

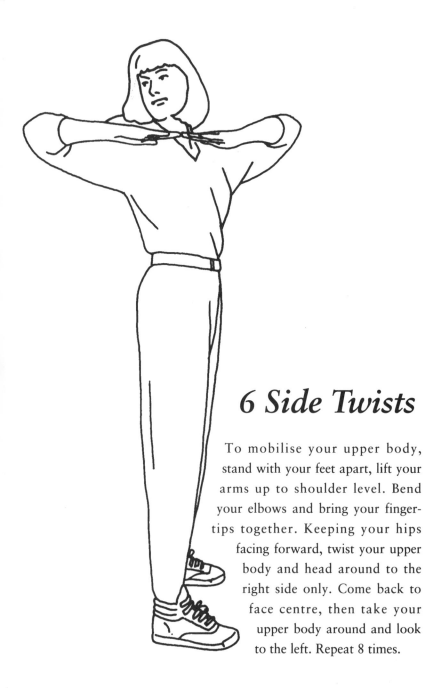

6 Side Twists

To mobilise your upper body, stand with your feet apart, lift your arms up to shoulder level. Bend your elbows and bring your fingertips together. Keeping your hips facing forward, twist your upper body and head around to the right side only. Come back to face centre, then take your upper body around and look to the left. Repeat 8 times.

7 *Side Reaches*

To mobilise the sides of your body, stand with your feet apart and knees relaxed. With your right arm, reach up and over your head, bending your left knee. Bring your arm down and transfer your weight on to your right leg and reach up and over with your left hand, as if you are climbing up a rope. Repeat 8 times to alternate sides.

WARM-UP STRETCHES

All stretches should be performed smoothly and held for 2–8 seconds. Do not bounce.

8 Calf Stretch

To stretch out the back of the lower leg, face a wall or tree for support. Stand with feet hip-width apart, toes facing forward. Place your hands up on a wall or solid support at shoulder level. Keep your arms straight, bend your left knee and take your right foot back further behind you. Keep your right leg straight and press your heel down until you feel the stretch in your right calf. Hold for 2–8 seconds, then repeat with the left leg.

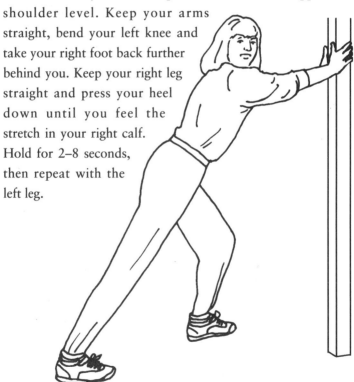

9 *Hamstring Stretch*

To stretch out the back of thigh and bottom, stand with your right foot back as before, but take your left foot forward, place heel down and toes up against a tree, wall or other support. Hold on to support at shoulder level, keep both knees straight, bend your arms and incline your body forward until you feel the stretch in the back of your upper left thigh and bottom. Hold for 2–8 seconds, then repeat with your other leg.

Alternatively, you may find it more comfortable to hold on to the support and with your back leg straight, bend the knee of your front leg and place your foot up on a small bench or step, approximately 4 inches off the ground (see illustration). Incline forward slightly. (See also the seated alternative – exercise 38, page 71.)

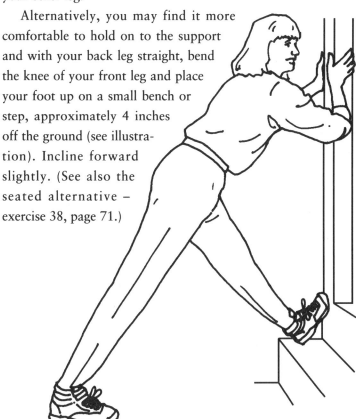

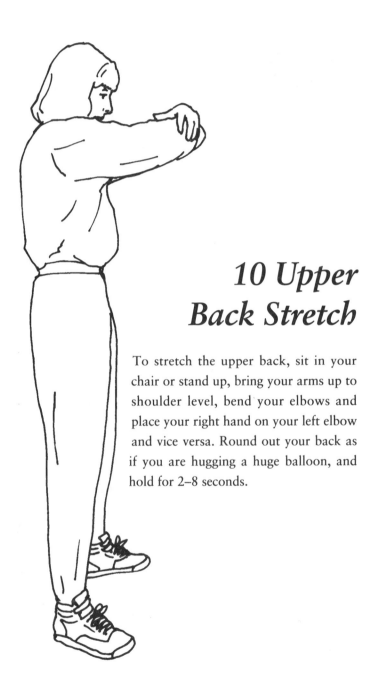

10 Upper Back Stretch

To stretch the upper back, sit in your chair or stand up, bring your arms up to shoulder level, bend your elbows and place your right hand on your left elbow and vice versa. Round out your back as if you are hugging a huge balloon, and hold for 2–8 seconds.

11 Triceps Stretch

To stretch out the back of your upper arm, sit or stand, take your right arm up and place your right hand behind your neck at shoulder level. Take your left hand across your chest and ease your right upper arm and shoulder back as far as comfortable. Hold for 2–8 seconds and repeat with the left arm.

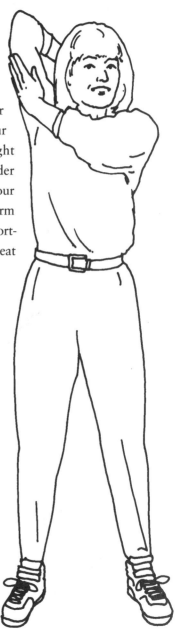

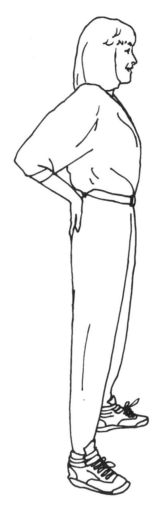

12 Chest Stretch

Sit forward on your chair or stand up, take both hands behind you and place them on your bottom. Pull your shoulders and elbows back, lift your rib cage up and feel the stretch across your chest. Hold for 2–8 seconds.

BONE BOOSTERS: AEROBICS

With our bodies warm and muscles prepared, it's time to concentrate on strengthening our heart (it's a muscle too). Regular exercise can improve heart and lung function and help control high blood-pressure. Blood-pressure changes with age and can increase through illness and over-exertion. Don't suddenly start to exercise if you already suffer from high blood-pressure – seek your doctor's advice first.

Blood-pressure is a measurement of the blood vessels during the heart's contractions and is measured using a sphygno-manometer. Two measurements are recorded: the lowest – when the heart is relaxed – is called the **diastolic** pressure and the highest – at the peak of contraction – is called the **systolic** pressure.

During our aerobic section, the aim of the exercises are to raise the pulse by making the heart beat faster and to maintain this higher rate for a specific length of time in order to strengthen the heart and increase stamina. But increasing the heart rate too fast, and for too long, can cause undue strain so the length of time must be varied according to age and ability.

Before you make a start on this section for the first time, observe how hard you need to work to achieve this. There are several ways you can do it. Athletes and serious exercisers wear heart-rate monitors to tell them their exact heart rate when they train or work out. In order to find out your safe and effective training zone the scientific way, sit down and take your pulse by pressing your carotid artery – which can be found in the side of your neck – with the tips of your third and fourth fingers. Alternatively, press your radial artery on the outside of your wrist just below your thumb.

Use a digital watch, or clock with a second hand, and count the number of beats for 1 minute. What you are feeling is the systolic pressure peak: this is your resting heart rate. Now jog on the spot for 1 minute, stop, and immediately take your pulse again. This figure indicates your working heart rate. A rough guide to a normal/average pulse rate, appropriate to age, can be worked out by simply taking the figure of 220 beats per minute and subtracting your age.

For example:

Age	Average pulse rate
220 bpm for 30-year-old	190 bpm
220 bpm for 40-year-old	180 bpm
220 bpm for 50-year-old	170 bpm

The pulse rate at which you should exercise is called your 'personal training zone' and can now be calculated.

Generally speaking, until the age of 50, this zone should be between 60% and 85% of the age-related, average pulse rate; after 50, between 60% and 75%.

It will, of course, vary from one individual to another. People who are less fit may find that working at under 55% is an effort and that 75% or 85% is a difficult goal, while the more fit will need to work longer at the higher rate to gain any benefit. But even working at below 55% of the personal training zone will help improve general fitness.

Calculation of % Heart Rate

30-year-old:

Maximum heart rate	= 220 − age = 190
60%	= 190 x 0.6 = 114
80%	= 190 x 0.8 = 152

In the aerobic section we raise the pulse rate for several minutes. Over the months, we gradually aim to work out at this higher rate for 20 minutes in order to gain cardiovascular benefit. The over-50s should aim for 6–15 minutes at the raised rate, according to individual fitness and age.

The following age-related chart gives an indication of the aerobic training zone in which we need to exercise:

Target Heart Rate Zone			
	Estimated Maximum Heart Rate	60%–85% of Maximum	
Age		Beats Per Minute	Beats Per 10 Seconds
20	200	120–170	20–38
25	195	117–166	20–28
30	190	114–162	19–27
35	185	111–157	19–26
40	180	108–153	18–26
45	175	105–149	18–25
50	170	102–143	17–24
55	165	99–140	17–23
60	160	96–136	16–23
65	155	93–132	16–22
70	150	90–128	15–21
75	145	87–123	15–21
80	140	84–119	14–20

So, from the chart, an average 40-year-old's safe and effective training zone is between 108 and 153 beats per minute. It is possible to work within a safe training zone without taking your pulse – by perceiving your personal rate of exertion during exercise through simply listening to your body. Jog on the spot for a minute, then stop, and ask yourself how you feel – give yourself ratings.

For example:
1. Feel exhausted
2. Feel OK, but a bit 'puffed'
3. Feel good and could work harder

These are your individual perceived rates of exertion. Be aware of your body and ask yourself repeatedly during your work out: which level of fitness am I working at? If it is level 3, challenge yourself a bit more, build up the duration and intensity. If you feel uncomfortable and are breathless, in pain, or lack co-ordination, then decrease the duration and intensity to level 2. If you are experiencing level 1, take it easy but try to gradually build up over the following days and weeks until you feel a comfortable 2 or maybe, eventually, 3. Monitor your progress but don't overdo it.

The Borg scale (named after the first physiologist who identified that physical exertion is closely related to exercise intensity) shown on the next page is a more detailed form of PRE (Perceived Rate of Exertion) used by exercise professionals. The rating of PRE scale runs from 6 to 20 and is supposed to reflect heart rates ranging from 60 to 200 bpm (beats per minute). That is, if a person exercising feels that exercise is somewhat hard and gives it a rating of 13, multiplying this by 10 would give and equivalent heart rate of

130 bpm. This is based on a maximum heart rate of 200 bpm which will not be the same for everyone.

'Aerobics' mean exercising with air, and should cause you to puff a bit and breathe deeply. The increased intake of air will enable your muscles to work harder and for longer, resulting in increased stamina and improved heart and lung efficiency, as mentioned earlier. Aerobics are bone boosters for the spine, hips and ankles. To benefit, you should begin by exercising for 4 minutes, but aim to build up to the recommended 20 minutes of aerobic exercise in each session over the weeks. Try to exercise 3 times a week.

Perceived Rate of Exertion Scale		
PRE	Description	Heart rate equivalent
6		60 bpm
7	Very, very light	70 bpm
8		80 bpm
9	Very light	90 bpm
10		100 bpm
11	Fairly light	110 bpm
12		120 bpm
13	Somewhat hard	130 bpm
14		140 bpm
15	Hard	150 bpm
16		160 bpm
17	Very hard	170 bpm
18		180 bpm
19	Very, very hard	190 bpm
20		200 bpm

13 Aerobic March

Clear a space and put on some motivating music with a strong beat, then simply walk on the spot in time to it. Lift up your feet and roll through the ball of your foot, keeping your weight over your big and second toe. Continue for one minute, but keep breathing easily throughout. Lift your knees higher, pump your arms and march around the room or garden for another minute, to increase your circulation. You should begin to puff a bit.

14 Aerobic Stands

March to an upright chair (preferably without arms) and sit on the edge with your legs back and feet on the floor. Simply stand upright and sit back down again, without using your hands to push off. Repeat standing and sitting 10 times. Aim to stand up leading with your chest forward and hands on your thighs. This gets more difficult with age, especially if posture is bad and the shoulders rounded.

If this is the case, place your hands on a table in front to steady you. (It's important to correct posture and strengthen thighs in order to maintain physical independence into older age.)

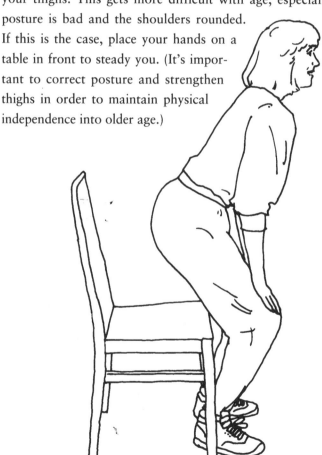

15 Aerobic Steps

March to a wide, dry stair or step with a non-slip surface, 4–6 inches high (8 inches if you are very fit). Stand facing it, but hold on to a banister or wall for support. Leading with your right heel, place your right foot up in the centre of the step. Make certain your body weight is over your knee and foot, and step up. Remember your posture. Stand tall. (Don't let heel or toe hang over the edge of the step.) Step your left foot up to join your right foot, leaning from the ankle joint. With your right foot, step back down, but keep close to the step and land on the ball of your foot, lowering your heel down to absorb the shock. Step back down with the left foot. Continue 'stepping' up and down for 1 minute. Change feet, and leading with the left foot, continue stepping for a further minute. (Try keeping in time to music.)

When your balance and skill have been achieved, do this stepping exercise without holding a support in order to maximise effect.

16 Aerobic Taps

Stand with feet together. Take your right foot out to the side and transfer your weight on to it. Bring your left foot across and tap it to the side of your right foot. Step with your left foot out to the side, transfer your weight on to it, and bring your right foot across and tap it to the side of your left foot. Continue stepping and tapping to the beat for 2 minutes. Increase the intensity by lifting your feet higher and stepping wider. Swing your arms and clap to the beat. The higher you swing, the more effective the exercise. Have fun and enjoy the rhythm.

When 90 young men immobilised in bed from 5–36 weeks were examined, they were found to be losing 5% of bone mineral content a month. Both bone and muscle strength gradually returned with normal activity. The bed-bound lose less if they get up every so often, and standing gives greater benefit than sitting. One piece of research showed that healthy young males alternating bed rest with 'quiet standing' for 2–4 hours reversed the bone loss.

17 Spot Walking

Gradually bring the intensity down. Just move in time to the music, walking on the spot for 1 minute with your hands at your sides. Return your body to its pre-aerobic state by placing your hands on your hips and simply transferring your weight from one foot to the other by lifting the heels only and keeping both feet in contact with the floor for another minute.

If your stamina is very low, it is important to build up this aerobic section gradually. You should feel 'puffed' but not exhausted, and you should be able to talk whilst you exercise. If your posture is poor, breathing is more difficult and the amount of air inhaled is less. For this reason, it is very important to maintain strength and mobility of the chest joints as we get older.

Low impact aerobic exercises have sufficient pull on the muscles to improve bone density of the lower limbs as well as to improve stamina.

BONE BOOSTERS: THE STRENGTHENERS

This unique Bone-Boosting section concentrates on exercises especially designed to strengthen the specific bones most vulnerable to osteoporotic fractures – the wrists, hips and spine. Many of the weight-bearing exercises are designed to put an extra stress on the bone and to strengthen the muscles supporting the bone, encouraging better balance and posture.

For Bone-Boosting to be effective, you need to gradually increase the number of repetitions during each session. The movements should be different to those bodily movements which you generally perform, and should stress, twist and bend your bones.

Stretching out the body is an important part of our life plan. Careful stretching of muscles maintains and increases flexibility, allowing our joints a full range of movement. This enables us to perform everyday tasks, like reaching for the top shelf, bending down to put on our shoes, or twisting round to pull up zips or fasten seat belts. But take care not to over-stretch at first. Listen to your body and hold the stretches for 2–4 seconds, gradually increasing to 8 or more only when you are comfortable. Back stretching exercises help decrease the curvature of the spine. But take care: forward bending exercises can make the problem worse.

Don't try to do everything in this section in one go. Concentrate on several of the exercises one day, and others the next, and gradually increase the length and intensity of your workout.

Throughout the exercises it is important to breathe correctly. Breathe out on effort and back in as you relax.

<u>Wrists, Arms and Shoulders</u>

18 Palm Presses

Sitting in your chair or standing, bring arms up to shoulder level, elbows bent. Place fingertips together in front of your chest. Push wrists together as hard as possible. Keeping your fingertips touching, open and close 12 times. You can do this and the following palm squeezes even whilst watching the TV.

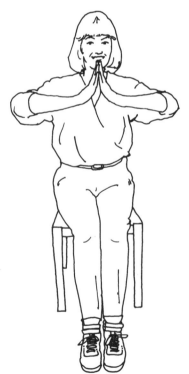

> *Are you right-handed? No prizes for guessing which of your arms is the stronger. When measured by bone scanners, upper arm bones of male baseball players aged between 8 and 19 showed a difference in strength according to the arm used. So did those of professional tennis players.*

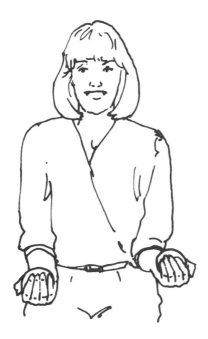

19 Palm Squeezes

Stand or sit to strengthen your wrists. Tuck your elbows into your waist. Lower your arms down out in front with your palms uppermost. Hold a soft ball or tennis ball in each hand. Squeeze as tightly as you can 12 times, keeping your arms and wrists steady.

20 Wind Ups

To strengthen your wrists and arms you need a stick or a pole an inch thick and 1–2 feet long. Tie a length of string 2–3 feet long in the centre of the pole, and tie a heavy object (a small plastic mineral water bottle, for instance) on to the other end.

Hold the stick at both ends, palms facing downwards, and wind up the string with a twisting action. Reverse the action, hold the stick palms upward and unwind. Do this exercise 4 times.

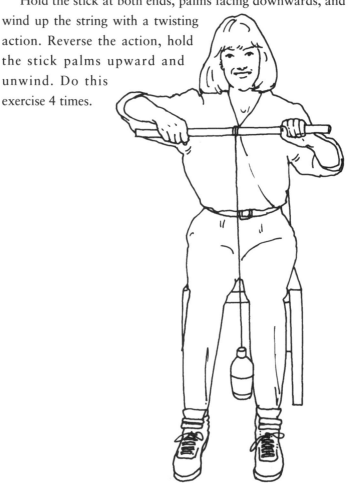

21 Lift Offs

Sit in an armchair and extend your legs in front of you, heels to the ground. Place your hands, fingers facing forward, flat on the arms of the chair. Incline your chest forward to correct your centre of gravity, take your weight on to your hands and keeping your legs straight, lift your bottom up and lower it back down 12 times. (Only a small lift is required.)

Alternatively, if you find this exercise difficult at first, sit further back on your seat. With your knees bent and hands on the arm of your chair, simply lift and lower your bottom. Gradually, in easy stages, sit forward on your seat, and straighten your legs as you lift and lower.

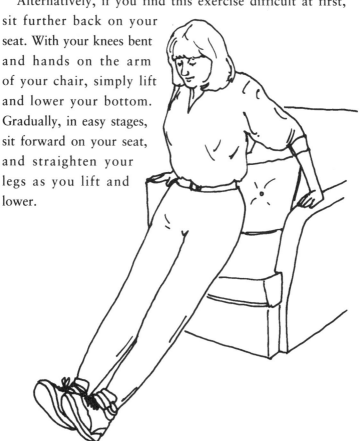

22 Push Aways

Stand with your legs comfortably apart, at least a foot away from a wall, with arms outstretched, shoulder width apart. Hands should be at shoulder level and fingers inclined inwards. Bend your elbows out, pull in your tummy and with a straight back, lower yourself towards the wall as far as comfortable, and press back up again. Repeat 8 times. (Don't allow your body to sag.)

This exercise is a beneficial Bone Booster with heels up, but with heels down, you can stretch out your calf muscles at the same time.

23 Pull Aways

To stretch out your arms, shoulders and spine, stand feet apart, a foot away from a secure kitchen sink unit or the banisters. Hold on with both hands, and keeping your legs straight, incline your upper body forward and take your weight on to your arms and shoulders. Drop your head between your arms, flatten out your back and hold for 2–8 seconds (23a). Bend your elbows, pull yourself up, step your right foot forward and bring your left foot to join it,

(a)

standing upright on your toes and resting your hips against the support (23b). Lower your heels and take first your right foot then your left foot back as before, and repeat the whole exercise with a smooth flowing movement 4 times. Heel raises correct the body's centre of gravity and improve balance.

(b)

24 Towel Up

(a) For Arms and Wrists – stand with feet comfortably apart, and hold both ends of a small hand towel out in front of you at shoulder level. Pull both ends, and keeping the towel taut, lift it up and over behind your head. Return it up and over to the front. Repeat 8 times, pulling hard on both ends.

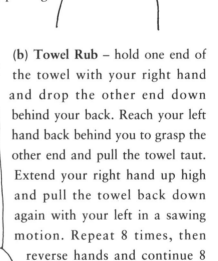

(b) Towel Rub – hold one end of the towel with your right hand and drop the other end down behind your back. Reach your left hand back behind you to grasp the other end and pull the towel taut. Extend your right hand up high and pull the towel back down again with your left in a sawing motion. Repeat 8 times, then reverse hands and continue 8 times to the other side.

Keep breathing naturally throughout these exercises. Don't hold your breath.

25 Shoulder Stretch

Sit down on the floor with your knees bent, feet apart and flat on the floor. Place your hands down behind your bottom, shoulder width apart, fingers facing forward. *Carefully* lift your bottom up, transferring weight on to your hands and push your chest forward. Hold for 2–4 seconds and lower back down. This stretch will also strengthen your arms and wrists.

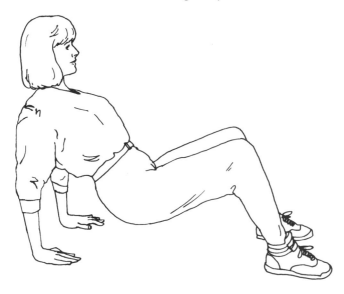

When nearly 100 elderly women practised squeezing a tennis ball for 30 seconds a day, they increased forearm bone density by up to 5.3% in just 6 weeks. Grip strength improved even more dramatically – up to 19% increase. But it was truly a case of losing it when not using it: a bone measure 6 months after the exercise routine stopped showed a loss of the previous gains.

Hips, Legs and Feet

26 Knees Over

Lie back on the floor, knees bent, feet flat on the floor. Hold a small weight or a 2 lb bag of sugar between your knees. Place your hands by the side of your bottom, palms facing down. Gripping the weight with your knees, roll your knees over to the right side as far as comfortable, keeping your feet in contact with the floor throughout this exercise. Bring knees back to centre and roll them over to the left. Repeat 4 times to each side, to strengthen hips and thighs.

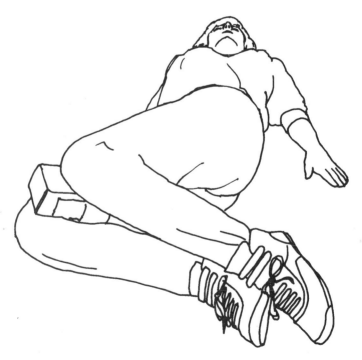

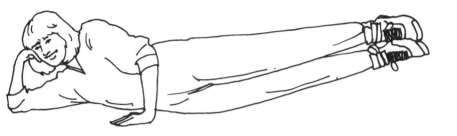

27 Leg Lifts

Lie on your right side, supporting your head with your right hand. Place your left hand on the floor in front of your waist for balance. Raise your left leg up approximately 12 inches and bring your right leg up to join it. Hold for 8 seconds, squeezing your thighs, knees, calves and ankles together. Relax and lower both legs down. Repeat 4 times to strengthen hips and spine. Roll over and exercise on your left side.

If you are new to exercise you may find this too advanced. Alternatively, lie on your right side as before, but bend your right leg and bring the knee forward to stabilise your position. Straighten and lift up your left leg only, hold it for 8 seconds and repeat 4 times. Roll over, bend your left leg and lift up your right leg. (Absolute beginners may find it more comfortable to begin by also bending the upper leg while lifting.)

28 *Fidgety & Edgy Feet*

(a) **Fidgety Feet** – stand with your feet comfortably apart, with hands on a garden fork or sweeping brush. Bend your knees inwards, take your weight on to your toes and push your heels out to the side. Place your weight back on your toes, push your knees out and bring your heels together. Repeat 12 times.

(b) **Edgy Feet** – place your feet wider apart, toes facing forward. To strengthen your ankles, bring your knees together and take your weight on your insteps. Keep feet parallel and body upright. Take your knees out wide and transfer your weight on to the sides of your feet. Repeat 12 times.

If you are not so stable on your feet, you can do these exercises sitting in a chair.

29 Hop It

One of the easiest and most effective ways to strengthen your ankles. Place your hands on your hips or hold on to the table worktop or banisters. Lift your left foot up behind you and simply hop 6 times on your right leg. Turn round, lift up your right foot behind you and hop 6 times on your left leg. To improve your balance, practise shutting your eyes while you hop, but stay close to the support, just in case! Repeat this exercise as often as possible. You could try doing it at the bus stop. Fellow travellers will only think you are impatient!

> *If all women past the menopause exercised regularly, the risk of hip fracture would be reduced by half, according to the British Medical Journal. That would mean around 20,000 fewer cases a year, which would spare a great deal of pain, money and hospital beds.*

30 *Quadriceps Stretch*

To stretch out the front of your thigh, stand with your feet together and with your left arm, hold on to a wall or unit. Bend your right leg and lift your foot up behind you, keeping both knees as close as you can. Take your right arm around and grasp your right ankle, easing your foot towards your bottom as far as is comfortable. Remember your posture – pull in your tummy, tuck your bottom under. Keep the front of your thighs parallel and feel the stretch. Hold for 2–8 seconds. Turn around and repeat with your left leg. To improve your balance, try doing this exercise without holding on to a support.

31 Hip Flexor Stretch

Stand with your feet together. Place your right foot out in front and bend your right knee. Take your left leg back as far as possible, heel up. Bend your right knee still further, lowering your body down until you feel a stretch in the front of your left hip. Keep your body upright and push the hip forward still further, and hold for 2–8 seconds. Try to keep your left knee straight. Repeat using the other side. If you find it difficult pushing away at low level, stand up a bit and push away from a higher level. But still tilt your hips forward and tuck your bottom under.

Women naturally have less leg power than men, so it stands to reason that by the age of 70, their legs will be weaker and they will be less mobile, relatively speaking. For this reason, it is most important to strengthen the quadriceps (the front thigh muscles), which are used for standing, walking and climbing up stairs. Strong muscles provide stability and support and, should a fall occur, help prevent breaks.

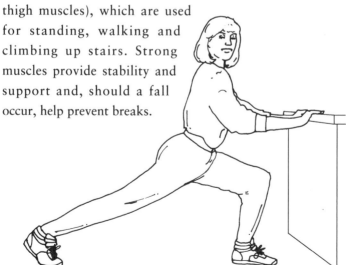

<u>Spine, Abdominals and Back</u>

Normal ageing shouldn't cause a person excessive loss of height, although a little is normal. However, with osteoporosis, the spinal discs collapse, resulting in poor posture, rounded shoulders, sunken chest and curvature of the spine. Poor posture is a major cause of immobility in older age.

If you already suffer from osteoporosis, do not attempt these exercises, but see our Osteo-Relief section (page 116) for alternatives.

32 *Chicken Neck*

To strengthen the upper spine and improve posture, sit in your chair or stand with your shoulders back down and relaxed. Fix your eyes on an object straight ahead. Keep your shoulders still, push your head forward and stick your chin out (**32a**). Keeping your chin parallel with the floor, pull it back in to your chest as far in as you can (**32b**). Try to keep your shoulders still and repeat these neck retractions for a minute. (A bit like a chicken!)

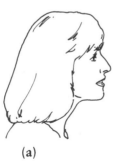
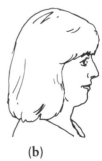

(a)   **(b)**

33 Ostrich Neck

Sit or stand as before and keep looking ahead. Stretch your neck and take your right ear over towards your right shoulder as far as is comfortable. Hold for 4 seconds, and take it back to centre. Take the left ear over to the left shoulder and hold for 4 seconds.

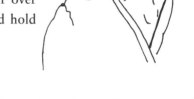

34 Spinal Lean

Stand with your right side close to a doorframe or secure high support. Hold on with your right hand at shoulder level. Take your left arm up and over your head to add extra weight and grasp the support. Keep your feet close in and with your legs straight, lean away from the support taking your weight out to the left side. Hold for 4 seconds. Lower your left arm and return to the upright position. Repeat 4 times, but don't lean forwards or backwards – that's cheating. Turn around and repeat 4 times to the other side.

35 *Spinal Twist*

Stand with your back a foot away from a wall unit or door frame, toes facing forward. Without moving your feet, twist your upper body around to the right only to hold the support. Hold for 2–4 seconds. (Keep hips facing the front.) Twist back to the front and on to the left side and hold. Repeat 4 times each side.

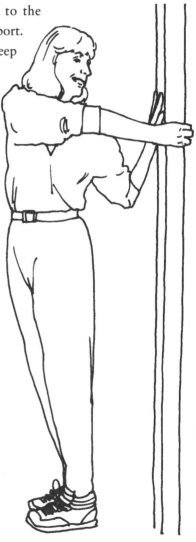

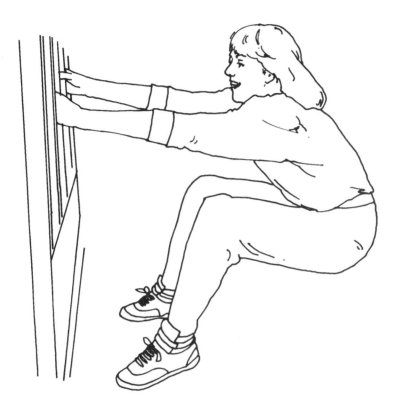

36 Spinal Reaches

To stretch out the shoulders and strengthen the spine, sit on the floor, knees bent, feet comfortably apart, facing a secure kitchen sink unit or banisters. Place your feet fairly close to the support. Reach up and grasp the edge. Using your arms and shoulders, pull up and lift your bottom off the ground. Hold 2–4 seconds and relax back down. Repeat 8 times. If you find this uncomfortably low, reach out and pull against something secure, but at a higher level.

37 *Push Backs*

A caved-in chest (inflexion) upsets the body's centre of gravity, and causes gait imbalance which can lead to falls. To counteract this, sit with your bottom well back in an upright chair which has a low back. Stretch out your arms and place hands, shoulder-width apart, on the edge of a table or desk in front of you. Bend your elbows out, round your back and slump forward. Straighten your arms, push back, lift up your rib cage and push your upper body back as far as possible over the back of the chair. Feel the stretch in your middle back. Repeat these movements 8 times. This simple but effective exercise improves posture and shoulder mobility, and assists correct breathing.

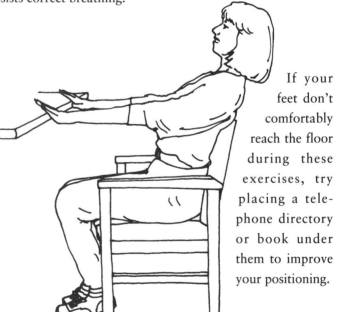

If your feet don't comfortably reach the floor during these exercises, try placing a telephone directory or book under them to improve your positioning.

38 Leg-Ups

To stretch out your lower spine and hamstrings, sit well back in an upright chair, knees bent, feet flat on the floor. Hold on to the back edge of your seat for support and lean your upper body forward, chest towards your knees. Straighten and lift your right leg (foot flexed, toes up), up to the level of your left knee. You should feel the stretch in your right hamstring and bottom. Hold for 2–4 seconds, relax down and repeat with your left leg. To encourage strength and flexibility, lift alternate legs 4 times. If you find this too difficult, keep the heel of your straight leg on the floor. Place your hands on your bent knee and lean your upright body forward, from the hips, until you feel the stretch in your hamstring.

When strengthening the spine, it is important to strengthen the abdominal muscles also, as these help support the spine. Therefore, first learn the pelvic tilt. Lie on your back, knees bent, feet flat on the floor. Pull in your tummy muscles, tilt your pelvis forward and push your lower back (waist) into the floor. This is the correct position for all abdominal work, and should be held throughout the following exercises.

39 *Tummy Trimmer One*

To strengthen the central abdominal muscles, place your hands on your thighs, then pelvic tilt, breathe out and lift your head and shoulders up off the floor to a count of 2. Breathe in and relax back down for a count of 2. Repeat 8 times, controlling both the up and down movement. (If your neck is uncomfortable, support the back of your head with one hand.)

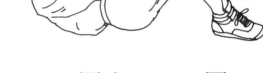

40 *Tummy Trimmer Two*

To strengthen the criss-cross abdominal muscles, from the same lying position, place your left arm, elbow bent, on the floor for support. Pelvic tilt, breathe out, lift your head and shoulders up to a count of 2, and with your right hand, twist across to touch your left knee. Breathe out and relax back down for a count of 2.

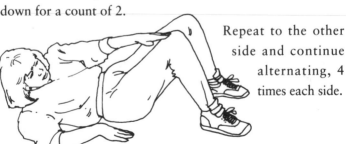

Repeat to the other side and continue alternating, 4 times each side.

41 The Flyer

Lie on your tummy with your chin on the floor. Bend your arms and place your elbows out to the sides at shoulder level, with hands forward and palms face down. Keep your head on the floor and pull your arms and shoulders back and up off the floor. Continue the exercise by lifting your head, chest and arms off the floor – keep them in a straight line – as if you are flying. Look down, don't throw your head back. Relax down, and repeat 8 times to strengthen your spine.

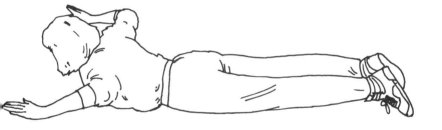

The floating weightlessness which astronauts experience in outer space may look like fun but has serious health consequences. The lack of stress on bones in the gravity-free environment causes bone loss to the tune of 2% for every month of flying time. To make up for it, pre-space training programmes include Bone-Booster exercises.

42 The Cat

To stretch out your spine, kneel up and place your hands on the floor under your shoulders, fingers facing forwards. Pull up your tummy muscles, drop your head down to look between your knees. Clench your buttocks and round and stretch out your back, like a cat does. Hold for 8 seconds. Relax back down, stick your bottom out and look up. Hold for 8 seconds, and relax.

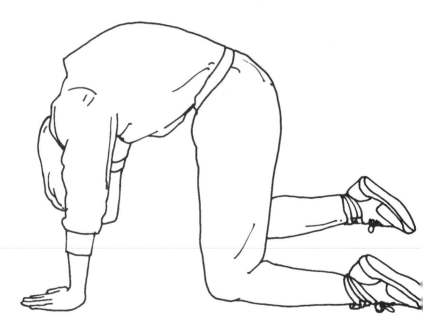

Relax and Remobility

Congratulations, you've almost finished! Get up in your own good time, and we'll kick start our bodies and get moving again.

Stand with your feet comfortably apart. Lift up your right knee and reach your left hand across and tap it on your knee. Lift your left knee and tap it with your right hand. Go on lifting and tapping 10 times. Finally, shake out your legs and your feet, then your arms and your hands.

The recent Carnegie Enquiry into the Third Age states: 'Appropriate exercise can delay or reverse physical decline and restore fitness among older people. Many people of between 50 and 74 are too unfit to benefit fully from the recent gains in years of life expectancy. If they moved about, walked and climbed stairs for a total of 60 minutes a day, they would be fitter, healthier and could enjoy a much more active and independent life-style.'

However, the good news is that if you stick to our *Bone Boosters* life plan and move dem bones, you will make them stronger and your body more resilient, by the constant but varied bending and stressing of the exercises which take the body through natural, but unexpected, movements. But to be effective they must be repeated regularly, ideally for 20–30 minutes, 3 times a week. So do your bones a favour and make exercise a part of your daily lifestyle.

WHICH SPORTS WORK BEST?

EXERCISE ROUTINES are not the only way to strengthen bones. You can also do this through various sports, dancing and physical activities. Unlike our 'designer' Bone Boosters, though, most sports don't give total-body protection, so we're not saying you can substitute, say, walking or jogging for our exercises. What we are saying is go ahead, enjoy as many ways as you can to keep fit and mobile – you'll have fun and know you're doing yourself a world of good.

Before we tell you about the best bone-preserving activities, we do have to remind you that bone-enhancing exercise is not always suitable for anyone with arthritis or heart disease, nor for anyone with established osteoporosis. (Remember, we've included a special chapter on this later in the book.) Talk to your doctor if in any doubt.

Why some sports are better than others

The key to strengthening bones is to put measured and controlled pressure on them. So it stands to reason that swimming, which is great for taking the pressure off joints, won't do much for the bones themselves. Of course, swimming is wonderful for increasing suppleness and mobility, and it increases muscular strength in the back, arms and legs too. But for bones, it's the short, sharp burst of activity you should go for; the kind that puts a momentary pressure on the bones, then releases, then repeats.

Put on your walking shoes

Around 20 minutes of brisk walking 3 times a week will provide the right amount of pressure to preserve bone in feet, legs, hips and lower spine, partly through the force of gravity, partly through muscular contraction. Walking is good for the heart and lungs, too, but does little for upper spine, neck and arms, so make sure you do our appropriate Bone Boosters too. You need to walk fast enough to feel a bit puffed, but not so out of breath that you can't say a few words to a companion. Wear shock-absorbing trainers, and invest in a pair of ankle-supporting walking shoes so you can keep up the routine in wet, wintry weather.

Running away with it

Running does all the things that walking does, only more so. It's tougher, of course, especially on the back, so if you feel the urge to start, take it slowly at first. You need good quality running shoes that will take the impact of hard and preferably softer surfaces – grass is better than pavements. Make sure you stretch leg muscles by using warm-up exercises for calf, hamstring (pages 36–37) and quadriceps (page 64) before you start. Begin by practising indoors running on the spot, limiting yourself to only 30 seconds a day if at first you find yourself getting breathless. Out of doors, expect to take at least 20 minutes to cover a mile daily for the first 6 weeks (the recommended rate for 40–50 age group). There's plenty of time to build up strength. Half an hour's running 3 times a week will keep you high in the fitness stakes. Always taper off slowly when you finish, don't just stop suddenly. This causes dizziness and can be harmful to your body.

Time for tennis .

Tennis makes a good alternative to running, but the game also provides bone-strengthening exercise for back, hips, legs, feet and wrists. And of course there's the heart/lung boost too, plus mobility for waist and shoulders. A couple of games a week plus Bone Boosters will do the trick.

Get rhythm

Dancing is more or less the equivalent of running or jogging, with the same kinds of benefits and limitations. Some dance routines include plenty of stretch – jazz dancing for instance – others, like tap or flamenco, provide more jogging-type impact. Make sure you go to a studio with a proper wooden-sprung floor. Dance can be tough on back and knees, and dance shoes don't provide cushioning to soften the impact. Look out for special 50-plus exercise-to-music classes, or a Medau whole-body movement class.

Golf benefits

An average 18-hole round is covered in a 4–5 mile walk, and that's the main gain to be had from golf. Not as good as ordinary walking, in fact, since those miles are likely to be covered at no more than a stroll – and that's assuming you don't hitch a lift on the golf trolley. Bonus for bones comes with increased grip strength from swinging that club. You also gain some flexibility in waist and hips. But don't depend on golf to keep your bones in good order.

Is cycling for softies?

Not if you include traffic dodging and inhaling petrol fumes! But apart from increased grip and arm strength, it's not great for bones, though you do get heart/lung exercise, knee flexibility and leg muscle enhancement. It's best to be gradual on this one – expect to start with 2 miles a day, 5 days a week, to be covered in 11 minutes if you're aged 40–50. And make sure you keep up your Bone Boosters.

Row the boat away

Yes, it's an ideal exercise for wrists and forearm bones. Not too practical for most people on a daily basis, but if you follow our *Bone Boosters* routine you'll be able to adapt to a pair of oars with ease. Indoors, a rowing machine is great for strengthening the abdominals but take care not to strain your back.

Hang on to your sailboard

Windsurfing puts stress on the wrists with its gripping action and when you pull on the sail, it strengthens your spine.

Great weight-training

This is the perfect work-out for bones. It gives short, sharp bursts of bone-loading movements. You can buy small weights with instructions for home use or use baked bean cans and plastic mineral water bottles straight out of the kitchen cupboard at no extra expense. Choose a variety of exercises to work arms, shoulders, back and legs. Work out 2–3 times a week.

Yoga – not just pretty poses

There are various yoga systems, the best for body movement being hatha yoga. The exercises systematically stretch muscles and put stress on joints and bones. They improve posture and help correct postural faults. Yoga is best undertaken in a class where a teacher can assess how much or how little

> *Exercise can make you feel sexy. A report on 8,000 women in Los Angeles revealed that a quarter of them felt an increase in sexual desire immediately after physical exercise. Long-term effects were even greater: 31% said they had more frequent sex once they began their exercise programme, 40% noted an increase in arousal and 25% experienced an increase in their ability to reach orgasm. All this for a minimum of 3 hours a week of moderate exercise such as tennis, walking, swimming or cycling.*

you can do. Some centres hold remedial classes for people with disabilities, arthritis, etc. Go for sessions at least twice a week.

Bowled over

Indoor or outdoor bowling is great for the wrists. You get the weight, the twist and the grip action.

Skate and ski

Gains: weight bearing on ankles and hips, grip and strike action for wrists, weight bearing, twists and turns for spine. Plus weight of ski boots! Losses: risk of falls and breaks (like Diana!).

It's not true that exercise only does you good if it hurts. Going for the burn is old hat, so is working up a heavy sweat. These excesses put a strain on the heart and could even be fatal for anyone unused to heavy exertion. A gentle start building up to greater endurance over weeks and months is the modern approach to sports and exercise. Never work yourself to the point of exhaustion; wear light clothing; take extra fluid if you find yourself getting thirsty; take a warm bath after vigorous exercising to ease muscles.

> *Sorry to mention it again, but the warm-up is important. Without a warm-up, you may suffer from cramp, a strained muscle, or even a heart attack. Warm-up for 5–10 minutes and always cool down gradually, don't stop suddenly.*

Hop, skip and jump

When you skip and hop, all body weight is on one leg. One of the most beneficial Bone Boosters.

Rubber-band workouts

These modestly-priced exercise bands can add resistance to many basic exercises. You can get them at local sports shops.

WHAT
WE NEED
TO EAT
AND WHY

OST OF US have the vague idea that we eat a reasonably healthy diet, without giving the subject too much thought. If we're fit, have enough energy, get few infections, we tend to take for granted that all is well. But sometimes we're missing more than we realise. A lifetime of watching weight, cutting down on dairy foods especially, can markedly diminish our intake of certain nutrients. We also have to remember that cooking reduces the vitamin and mineral content of our food. And sometimes what we buy is not as fresh as it might be, so again vitamins and minerals are reduced.

Certain lifestyles may require extra nutrients. If we smoke, drink, or use the contraceptive pill, we may need higher than the normal recommended intake of Vitamin C. A diet high in protein, particularly red meat, is thought to reduce the body's capacity to utilise calcium. A recent survey suggested that vegetarian, non-smoking women under 45 have lower-than-normal bone density in their hips, though only a small sample was studied and more research is needed. Certain drugs reduce the amount of vitamins and minerals that our bodies can utilise. The use of steroids, for instance, calls for a higher-than-normal intake of calcium and Vitamin D. And at all ages, but especially at the menopause, we need calcium.

Why is calcium special?

Bone tissue's main components are calcium and phosphorus, which are embedded in a framework of fibres made of collagen. Calcium gives bones strength and hardness. Phosphorus helps the body to absorb calcium, and collagen provides flexibility. Calcium is the one we have to watch. We need it before we are born, when our bones begin to form in the womb; we need it in infancy, when our bones are growing; and we need it in adulthood to maintain bone density. Almost all the calcium in our bodies is stored in bones, and is there to give strength and rigidity. We also have calcium in dentine, the hard substance out of which teeth are formed.

New bone continuously replaces old, and we need constant supplies of calcium to make that new bone healthy. One theory about the rise in osteoporosis in post-menopausal women is that they have not received sufficient calcium as

Alcohol taken in excess may be bad for bones, but in moderation it can be a positive help. Some recent research from America revealed that the bone strength of over 350 women and men improved over a span of 18 years, increasing with a rise in their alcohol consumption. The findings are being greeted with caution by most medics, but it's beginning to look as if a glass or two of wine a day are an aid to health, not a hazard, backing up other recent findings that show moderate alcohol intake is a protection against heart attacks and strokes.

children and throughout their young adult lives, and therefore their bone density is already lower than it should be at
the time of menopause. Another possibility is that bone loss is
accelerated more quickly than normal in those who have had
a low-calcium diet in earlier years. For this reason, watching
calcium intake is important throughout life as a way of
conserving bone.

Calcium and ageing

From about the age of 35, the bones begin to lose the ability
to replace high levels of calcium in new bone. The loss
normally remains gradual while the ovaries produce regular
amounts of oestrogen and the diet contains adequate
amounts of calcium. (It is the combination of oestrogen with
calcium that ensures bone strength.) But oestrogen production from the ovaries ceases at the menopause, which is why
bone loss increases then. In addition, older people absorb
vitamins and minerals less efficiently, so the amount of
calcium available is reduced.

Is extra calcium a protection during the menopause?

No one is quite sure how much protection extra calcium gives
once periods stop. One school of thought states that when
there's no oestrogen from the ovaries, taking extra calcium in
the diet or in supplements is of little use. But when HRT is

also taken, the story is different, since near-pre-menopausal oestrogen levels are restored and interact beneficially with calcium.

Even so, there are still ifs and buts, the main one being that the body does in fact still continue to store low levels of oestrogen in the adrenal glands, and there may still be some interaction with calcium. Most experts would play safe and recommend a diet that includes regular amounts of calcium daily after the menopause whether on HRT or not – see below for how much and which foods. There is also no doubt of the value of keeping up calcium intake in the years leading to the menopause.

The same question occurs about calcium and exercise: is extra calcium used to good effect in someone who does not exercise? Again the answer is not clear. There is some evidence that women who exercise and take extra calcium in their diet maintain or gain bone density, even in old age, but the evidence is not conclusive. Doing both makes the most sense.

How much calcium is needed?

In recent years, the recommended daily allowance (RDA) has been upped to reflect changes in scientific thinking. Even so, opinion differs as to how much calcium we need, and its combination with Vitamin D may be as important a factor as raising levels of calcium alone – see more on this below. Recommended daily allowances of calcium are based on the needs of the population at large and not on individuals who may have special requirements because of their lifestyle or dietary habits. The amounts differ according to age. We're giving figures recommended by the National Osteoporosis Society which are higher than those given by other recognised authorities.

Children aged 12 and under	800 mg
People aged 13–19	1,200 mg
Adults: Women aged 20–40 and men aged 20–60	1,000 mg
Pregnant and nursing women	1,200 mg
Women over 40	1,500 mg
Men and women over 60	1,200 mg

(Nobody should exceed 2,000 mg a day.)

Which foods provide this?

Milk, cheese and dairy products are the best source of calcium, also oily and canned fish, dark green vegetables, nuts and dried fruit. There is very little calcium in meat, not much in lentils or similar dried pulses. Low-fat foods can be as good a source of calcium as full fat ones, if not better – see skimmed milk. Here are a few common foods with high calcium content (in mg). For a comprehensive list, see CALCIUM COUNTDOWN at the end of this section, on page 97.

half pint of silver-top whole milk	340 mg
half pint of skimmed milk	360 mg
small pot of low-fat yoghurt	225 mg
2 oz sardines	220 mg
4 oz canned pilchards	342 mg
2 oz cheddar cheese	415 mg

Are calcium supplements a good idea?

There's some controversy over this, but many doctors think that calcium supplements are worth taking as a way to help retain bone. It's even possible to get supplements on prescription. But extra calcium seems to help the elderly rather than those losing bone around the time of the menopause. There's quite a body of evidence showing that women in their 70s and older can even regain bone through taking extra calcium, but very little that's quite so encouraging for the 10 post-menopausal years. One study from America demonstrated that calcium supplementation significantly reduced bone loss in middle-aged women, particularly in the upper arm, but the research findings are not consistent, and it must be said that the medical profession disagrees over the issue. When calcium-enriched milk first came on to the market, the claims that it could protect against osteoporosis were fiercely challenged by doctors.

Even so, if you're not sure you can take sufficient calcium from ordinary foods, you might want to try supplements. There are various kinds available from chemists with a recommended dose of from one to six or more tablets a day. Newest research suggests that calcium supplements are more effective when Vitamin D is added, and indeed this could be as important as calcium and physical activity in helping preserve bone density. You can buy combined calcium and Vitamin D supplements. Examine the label before you buy a supplement, and if necessary check with the chemist that you'll be getting around one gram of calcium a day since the amount made available to the body is not the same as the actual dose as stated on the pack. Soluble types are thought to be the most speedily absorbed, and you can also get kinds to chew or swallow whole. Sometimes calcium supplements cause constipation, if so, try another type. Some experts claim that they are best absorbed if taken at night.

Vitamin D – the necessary extra

We need Vitamin D in order to absorb calcium properly. But as we grow older, we become less able to utilise the vitamin, and a deficiency may lead to muscular weakness and contribute to instability, falls and subsequent fractures. Some drugs interfere with Vitamin D absorption. If you take any drug regularly, ask your doctor about this.

Main dietary sources of Vitamin D are oily fish like herring, sardine, mackerel; also egg yolk, milk, butter, cod liver oil. Some foods like breakfast cereals, margarines and

> *It's not fully proven, but there's some evidence that if you've had children you may be less susceptible to osteoporosis. The advantage may come from increased intake of calcium-rich foods, which many pregnant women include in their diet. Also, high levels of oestrogen during pregnancy boost Vitamin D productivity, which in turn promotes calcium absorption. And on top of all that, the hormone progesterone, which is present in higher levels in pregnancy, adds to the bone-conserving effect.*

skimmed milk powder are fortified with Vitamin D – if so, this will be stated on the pack. We also get Vitamin D from sunlight, which is why getting out into the fresh air in winter as well as summer is important, especially as we grow older and may give in to the temptation of staying indoors. Some calcium supplements include Vitamin D as the natural complement. It is generally better to take a combined supplement rather than trying Vitamin D alone, in order to get the right balance.

Magnesium – another part of the picture

The mineral magnesium is thought to help stabilise hormones that control calcium balance and can help increase the efficacy of Vitamin D. Western diets contain very variable amounts of magnesium, and there's a school of thought that supports increasing dietary intake of the mineral as a way to keep bones strong, especially if you are increasing calcium.

Orthodox medicine does not hold with the idea that we may be magnesium deficient, but it's as well to know which foods contain it. One of the best sources is cocoa, which means that it is also in chocolate, both milk and plain.

Other sources are wheat bran, nuts, tea and coffee, oats and rice. And it comes via the tap in drinking water – more in hard than in soft water – so make a habit of drinking several glasses a day.

And finally, phosphorus

This mineral also plays a part in calcium absorption and in the formation of tissue between bones. We get it in meat, poultry, fish, cereals, soft drinks, and it's highly unlikely that we get too little.

Is there a case for a multivitamin pill?

If you are concerned about receiving sufficient nutrients in your daily diet, the answer might be to go for a multivitamin pill that offers a balance of various vitamins and also minerals. You won't get as much calcium in a multi-pill as you do in calcium-only types, though. Look on the labels to compare contents. In any case, a vitamin pill is not an excuse to give up being concerned about what you eat. A balanced diet is important for general fitness and health, whatever supplements you take.

The good mid-life diet

- Reduce sugar, not only in tea and coffee, but by choosing natural, unsweetened fruit juice instead of canned soft drinks. And don't forget the sugar content of cakes, biscuits, puddings and jams.
- Reduce salt, both in cooking and when seasoning food at the table. Some salted foods need to be eaten sparingly: crisps, salted nuts, smoked fish, smoked bacon, smoked meats like salami.

- Eat vegetables and salads daily. Best is a combination of green, leafy vegetables, yellow and red vegetables, peas and beans for fibre content and uncooked salads. At least 3 helpings a day.
- Have fresh fruit daily. At least 2 servings.
- Go for fibre. You'll get it in cereals, and it's a way to make calcium-rich milk go down too, so try to eat at least one helping a day. Other fibre foods which can protect against heart disease and bowel disorders are bananas, avocado pears, celery, fresh fruit, lentils and other dried beans and pulses, and oatmeal. Remember, unprocessed bran can hinder calcium uptake, so avoid the stuff.
- Limit meat consumption. Red meat is best kept to 2 or 3 helpings a week; substitute chicken, fish, nuts as sources of protein.
- Limit fats and dairy products. To protect against heart disease, fat intake should be about a third of total calories consumed. Use olive, sunflower, safflower oils rather than animal fats for cooking, whether it's roasting, frying, or in salad dressings. Choose skimmed milk, low-fat yoghurts.
- Drink plenty of liquids. It can be water, up to 6 large glasses daily, or fruit juice, or herbal tea which is, of course, caffeine-free.
- Alcohol consumption should be limited. Maximum safe limit for women is 14 units a week, 1 unit being half a pint of beer or a small glass of wine or standard measure of spirits. Alcohol can cause flushes, and in excess hampers calcium absorption and damages bone cells, so drinking even less is better.

> *Keep down your coffee intake and don't take it black. An American study shows that drinking more than 2 cups a day appreciably reduces bone density, though women who also drank at least one glass of milk lost less bone than other coffee drinkers.*

- Smoking? As well as all the other horrors connected with smoking, it triggers an early menopause and is strongly associated with risk of fractures. Even passive smokers, women who live with heavy smokers, have been found to have an earlier-than-average menopause with risk of greater reduction of bone density. (See box on page 21.)

The fringe and beyond

Claims for various 'alternative' ways to combat osteoporosis make headlines from time to time, some of which are based on research, others merely on passionate conviction. A trace element called boron has been named as a vital ingredient in maintaining calcium levels and so reducing bone loss in post-menopausal women. The results seem impressive – calcium loss reduced by 50%, blood levels of oestrogen doubled in one report – but as is so often the case with alternative reme-dies, the number of women studied was very small, just a dozen, and more research is needed before claims can be justified. But boron exists in fruit such as apples and pears, in leafy vegetables and nuts, and is available at health food stores in tablet form, though most nutritionists wouldn't recommend buying it.

Yet another trace element, silica, is said to 'empower' calcium and therefore prevent osteoporosis, as well as strengthen nails and hair. The orthodox view is that we get enough in our diet, since silica is present in the earth, but the alternative view is that high-tech farming has destroyed it and modern food-processing removes what little is left. Brown rice, wholemeal flour, fresh fruit eaten with the peel intact and organically-grown products can provide silica.

Another branch of the alternative fringe, Chinese medicine, advocates herbal concoctions that act on the kidneys. Recent reports on possible kidney damage from Chinese treatments suggest that this one should be approached with great caution.

CALCIUM COUNTDOWN

The following is a comprehensive list of foods and the amounts of calcium they contain. We don't suggest you start weighing out and counting. Use the list as a rough check to get an idea of the calcium you get in your daily diet.

(Calcium per 100 g – approx 4 oz – unless otherwise stated; amounts are in mg, i.e. in 100 g of white flour there are 15 mg of calcium.)

Flour, bread and cereals

Flour, white	15
wholemeal	35
fortified, white	140
fortified, brown	150
self-raising *(depending on raising agent)*	350
Bread, one large slice, white or wholemeal, fortified	60
Rolls, brown or white	120
Albran	74
Cornflakes	3
Muesli	200
Oatmeal in porridge	6
Puffed wheat	26
Ready Brek	64
Rice Krispies	7
Shredded Wheat	38
Special K	42

Sugar Puffs	14
Weetabix	33
Macaroni, boiled	8
Rice, boiled	1
Spaghetti, boiled	7
canned in tomato sauce	21

Biscuits, cake, puddings

Chocolate biscuit	110
Digestive biscuit	110
Fruit cake	75
Ginger biscuit	130
Jam tart	62
Pastry	110
Shortbread	97
Sponge cake	140
Water biscuit	120

Dairy foods

Butter	15
Cheese, Camembert	380
Cheddar	800
Edam	740
Parmesan	1,220
Stilton	360
Cottage	60
Cream cheese	98
Condensed milk	280
Cream, double	50
Custard, egg	130
with powder	140

Egg, size 2	40
Evaporated milk	280
Fromage frais, 250 g pot	244
Goat's milk	130
Ice cream, dairy	140
Milk, half pint, silver-top	340
half pint, skimmed	360
Yoghurt, small pot, low fat	225

Fish

Cod, baked	22
Fish fingers, fried	45
Haddock, fried in batter	110
smoked	58
Halibut, steamed	13
Herring, grilled	43
Mackerel, fried	28
Pilchards, in tomato sauce	300
Plaice or sole, fried in batter	93
Prawns	150
Salmon, poached	29
canned	93
smoked	19
Sardines, in oil	550
Scampi, fried	99
Trout, poached	24
Tuna, canned	7

Meat

Bacon, fried rasher	16
Beef, minced, stewed	18
roast	6

Beefburger, fried	33
Chicken, duck, turkey, roast (*average*)	11
Corned beef	14
Ham	9
Lamb, grilled or roast	9
Liver, fried	15
Pork, grilled or roast	10
Sausages, pork, grilled	53
frankfurter	34
Veal cutlet, fried	14

Vegetables

Asparagus, boiled	13
Aubergine, raw	10
Butter beans, boiled	19
Baked beans, canned in tomato sauce	45
Beetroot	30
Broccoli	46
Brussels sprouts	25
Cabbage, boiled	53
Carrots, boiled	37
Cauliflower, boiled	18
Celery, raw	52
Chickpeas, boiled	64
Cucumber	44
French beans, boiled	39
Leeks, boiled	61
Lentils, boiled	13
Lettuce	23
Mushrooms, fried	4
Onions, fried	61
Parsley, raw	330
Parsnips, boiled	36

Peas, frozen, boiled	31
canned	24
Pepper, green, raw	9
Potatoes, boiled	4
baked or roast	12
chipped	14
Spinach, boiled *	600 (*170 utilized*)
Spring greens, boiled	86
Swede, boiled	42
Sweet corn, on cob, boiled	4
canned	3
Tomatoes, raw	13
Turnips, boiled	55
Watercress, raw	220

(*Absorption of calcium is impaired in some foods, i.e. spinach and other vegetables, or is lost during heating or cooking although amounts are still high.)

Fruit

Apples	4
Apricots, fresh	16
dried	104
Banana	7
Blackberries, raw	63
Cherries	16
Dates, dried	58
Gooseberries	28
Grapes, black	4
white	19
Grapefruit	17
Melon	9
Orange	41
Peach	5

Pear	8
Pineapple, fresh or canned	12
Plums	14
Prunes, stewed	17
Raisins	61
Raspberries	41
Rhubarb	84
Strawberries	22
Sultanas	52
Tangerines	42

Nuts

Almonds	250
Brazils	180
Peanuts	61
Walnuts	61

Oils and fats

Cod liver oil	*trace*
Lard	1
Margarine, low-fat	*trace*
other	4
Vegetable oil	*trace*

Sugar and jams

Sugar, demerara	53
white	2
Honey	8
Jam	24
Marmalade	45

Drinks

Drinking chocolate	33
Cocoa powder	130
Coffee, roasted	120
infused	122
instant	160
Tea, Indian	430
infused	*trace*
Coca-Cola	4
Fruit juice, canned	10
Lemonade	5
Lucozade	5
Orange juice, fresh	12

Alcohol

Beer	8
Lager	4
Cider	8
Wine, red	7
white	9

To get around 1,200 to 1,500 mg of calcium from a daily diet, as a rough guide you'd need to have at least two thirds of a pint of milk, take some of it in morning cereal, also in tea and coffee. Plus a pot of yogurt or fromage frais or 1 oz of cheddar cheese, four slices of bread, two helpings of dark green vegetables, two pieces of fruit. This adds up to over 1,000 mg, and the rest can be derived from fish, nuts, dried fruit, eggs, etc. Don't forget that you get extra calcium when you add grated cheese to dishes, or yoghurt to soups. Eat the bones in canned fish like sardines and pilchards to get the full calcium content.

OSTEOPOROSIS

The medical treatments

Though HRT, hormone replacement therapy, steals the headlines, there are several other new drug treatments for osteoporosis which can prevent or restore bone loss. There's even a variation of HRT that can eliminate the artificial 'breakthrough' periods you get with standard HRT. Here's a summary of the treatments available.

EVERYTHING YOU NEED TO KNOW ABOUT TAKING HRT

The replacement hormone is, of course, oestrogen. It not only helps retain bone strength, it also reduces or eliminates hot flushes, vaginal dryness and other temporary menopausal symptoms, and it may also strengthen muscle tone. Though oestrogen has been used to treat the menopause for at least 30 years, it has been widely available only within the last 10 years. Therefore, despite its excellent track record, there are no really long-term, large-scale studies of its effects. Until the early 1980s, oestrogen alone was given. Then an increase in cases of endometrial cancer came to light (this is cancer of the womb lining) and so a second important female hormone, progestogen, was included to induce a monthly shedding of the womb lining in order to minimise the cancer risk. Now, every woman on HRT gets the combined version except, logically enough, those who have had a hysterectomy.

The more recent worry with HRT is a slightly increased risk of breast cancer. There is no risk in fact when it is taken for 5 years, a possible very, very slight risk if taken for 10 years, and a small but clear statistical risk if taken for longer than 10 years. That is why a careful health check should be made at the start of taking HRT, with 6-monthly checks afterwards, and monthly self-examination of breasts. Around 60–70% of women on HRT take it for less than a year, many giving up for fear of cancer or through dislike of the break-through periods. In the UK, only 8–10% of menopausal women are on HRT; in the US, it's 80%.

How long should HRT be taken to protect bones?

Some doctors recommend taking it for life from the onset of the menopause, which perhaps shows more enthusiasm than prudence given our present knowledge. The general consensus is 5–10 years. The treatment works best up to the age of 65.

When is the best time to start?

The time when most bone loss occurs is 10 years from the date of the last period. Some doctors advise starting on HRT straight away, or even before periods stop if there's any pre-menopausal sign of bone loss. A more moderate recommendation is to start within a couple of years of the menopause.

Will HRT restore bone?

This is another issue the medics don't agree on. Some claim HRT can restore bone in spine and thigh after a year of treatment. Others say that it's collagen, a substance affecting skin thickness, that appears to increase. The general consensus in the medical profession is that HRT can only prevent further loss. And once the treatment is stopped, bone loss resumes at the former rate. Other menopausal symptoms may also reappear when the treatment stops.

Is it safe to take HRT after an early menopause, including after hysterectomy?

Women who have had their ovaries removed in, say, their 30s, can get hot flushes as well as the kind of bone loss associated with women 10–15 years their senior. Even when ovaries are intact after hysterectomy, they are likely to stop producing oestrogen within 2–4 years. If you've had a hysterectomy, with or without ovaries removed, ask for a bone screening.

Who shouldn't take HRT?

Opinions on this vary too. We can only give you the facts and the limits of current knowledge. Some specialists will happily prescribe HRT to women who have had breast or endometrial (womb lining) cancer, or other forms of cancer. Many doctors, however, will be more cautious and weigh the comparative risk of stimulating new tumours against that of suffering severe fractures in the individual they are treating. Similar doubts play a part for women with a mother or sister who has had breast cancer, and who are therefore known to be at risk. There's also a question mark about HRT after benign breast disease – non-malignant lumps or cysts. No one yet knows the risks of taking HRT for 10 years for such women. Gall bladder and liver disease, a history of blood-clotting, epilepsy or kidney problems, diabetes or fibroids may also mean that HRT is not suitable. On the other hand, HRT is safe for anyone with high blood-pressure – it may even cause a healthy decrease in levels. If you are in doubt, ask to see a full fact sheet and discuss the matter with your doctor.

How is the treatment given?

It can be in the form of pills or a transdermal patch, which is simply a hormone-loaded plaster attached to an area of the buttocks or abdomen, which is replaced every few days. A third method of delivery is a slow-release implant, a pellet inserted into the abdomen with effect for several months. That may not be so good if you find you suffer unwelcome side-effects. Also, implants can create a dependency on the treatment with increasing need for booster doses. Anyone who has had a hysterectomy will get any of these versions as unopposed oestrogen, since there is no danger of endometrial cancer. Everyone else, including women who've had one of the new ablation-methods now available as an alternative to hysterectomy, will be prescribed the hormone combination of oestrogen and progestogen. The combined treatment causes monthly breakthrough bleeding, the equivalent of a mild period lasting 2 or 3 days.

The latest variation on HRT is a version that will not cause breakthrough bleeding but will help reduce mood swings associated with the monthly period.

Are there any side-effects?

Breast tenderness, bloating and weight gain are the most common side-effects, followed by headaches, dizziness and gastric upsets. It's also possible to develop eye irritation, such as contact lens intolerance, skin rashes, brown skin patches, enlarged fibroids and facial hair, in which case the answer might be to forget HRT. With the more common symptoms, the usual advice is to carry on and see what happens, and in

HRT – the not-so-good news

Recent research suggests that HRT preserves bone only when taken for at least 7–9 years. The study, based on long-term observation, showed that as soon as women stopped taking it, their bone density declined rapidly. By the age of 75, their levels were only 3–5% higher than in women who had never taken hormone replacement.

many cases they disappear in two or three months. The other solution is to try another brand, since several pharmaceutical companies produce versions of HRT. Side-effects are most likely to be caused by the oestrogen content, though progestogen can also cause breast tenderness, bloating and occasionally depression. Transdermal patches and implants bypass the liver and should produce fewer side-effects, though they can cause local skin irritation.

HRT and heart disease

Many studies show that HRT reduces the risk of heart disease in women by up to 50% if it is taken for 5 years – an impressive and important claim. The research is based mainly on women using unopposed higher-dose oestrogen, as prescribed 10 or more years ago. With added progestogen and lower doses of oestrogen, the protective effect could be reduced. At the present time no one knows. The newer methods of delivery, patches and implants, have lower-still oestrogen content and are less well absorbed, so they are likely to lose out on the protective effect. Again, there is no research available.

Variations on the theme

The male hormone testosterone is sometimes added to the HRT cocktail. Testosterone can increase energy levels and libido. It is often administered as an implant, and although side-effects are said to be rare, there have been disturbing accounts of body hair growth, voice deepening and even baldness! Testosterone may also cancel out the heart disease protection or even increase risk of heart disease – no one yet knows. The other big variation is called tibolone (manufactured under the name Livial). This particular hormone mix (a synthetic formula of the same hormones, different proportions, plus a small amount of male hormone) eliminates those irritating breakthrough periods. Again no one yet knows whether it can offer heart disease protection. Livial comes in tablet form and is not usually prescribed until one to two years after natural periods stop. These variations can trigger similar side-effects to those caused by HRT.

OTHER PROTECTION AND TREATMENTS

Biphosphonates are a group of drugs that reduce bone deterioration and restore small amounts of bone, too. The kind used for osteoporosis is called etidronate disodium (trade name Didronel). It is suitable for women and men with diagnosed osteoporosis who may have suffered fractures, and is taken in tablet form alternating with calcium supplements, sometimes in addition to HRT. A pack of Didronel consists of 14 tablets to be taken on consecutive days, followed by 76 days on calcium. Vitamin D supplements might be added.

The treatment is prescribed for a period of 3 years and research has shown that after the first year bone density rises steadily with a dramatic drop in fracture rate. The benefit may not continue beyond this time, and may even be reversed. Side-effects can be gastric upset, nausea and diarrhoea, but are short-lived because of the brief time the drug is taken. The tablets are recommended to be taken 2 hours before or after eating to help eliminate side-effects. Didronel has been prescribed for osteoporosis for only 6 years and needs regular monitoring, but the drug has a 10-year safety record in treating Paget's disease, another bone condition. It's not suitable for people with a history of kidney problems or colitis.

Calcitonin is produced by the thyroid gland to maintain levels of calcium and other minerals. Production declines as we get older, and the lower levels could contribute to osteoporosis, though at present this is no more than conjecture. What is proven is that a form of calcitonin derived from salmon will

> *A version of sodium bicarbonate, commonly used for stomach upsets, could reduce calcium loss and even restore bone in women past the menopause. The treatment may work by neutralising the calcium-leaching effect of a protein-rich diet but the research is still in its infancy and further trials are needed.*

preserve bone in women past the menopause and can restore small amounts of bone if taken for a year. Calcitonin, often combined with extra calcium, can be given to older women and men too who are diagnosed as having osteoporosis. For these patients it can also reduce pain from spinal fractures. Use of calcitonin has been held back because it has to be given by injection, though there have been successful trials with a nasal spray version. It's also more expensive than Didronel.

Vitamin D and calcium (again) have a protective role for older women. A recent report that set the medics talking showed that Vitamin D and calcium supplements reduced fractures and increased bone density in women aged from 70 upwards. The trial involved over 3,000 women living in nursing homes or sheltered housing, all able to walk though some needed a cane or frame. Half of the women were given daily supplements of Vitamin D (800 International Units) and calcium (1.2 g), and the other half got dummy pills. After 18 months, the women on supplements had 43% fewer hip fractures and 32% fewer wrist or forearm fractures than those on the dummy-pills. The treated group also had a 2.7% increase in thigh bone density while the untreated group had a 4.6% decrease. There were gastric upsets in some of the 'takers', but no serious side-effects. One reason for the results could be that the women had a diet low in calcium and Vitamin D to start with. The trial took place in France, where dairy products are not fortified with vitamin D as they are in the UK. All the same, supplements instead of drugs could be beneficial for older women.

Fluoride can increase bone density, though it can also, in high amounts, increase risk of hip fractures. It's not available on prescription, but is offered in some specialist clinics to patients with very severe osteoporosis of the spine, perhaps combined with calcitonin and/or calcium. Side-effects may not be acceptable – gastrointestinal bleeding, leg pains, nausea – and in some cases, fractures have occurred even when bone density has improved, which could mean that it produces low-quality bone replacement.

Hormone replacement therapy can preserve muscle strength. Research from University College, London, has revealed that women's muscle strength can decline dramatically after the menopause. This may contribute to increased risk of falls and fractures. Now University College's physiology department is observing women on HRT and finding that the treatment not only seems to prevent muscle weakening but may also reverse low muscle strength.

Anabolic steroids can improve bone and muscle in older people, but the side-effects are even more daunting – extra body or facial hair, deepened voice, fluid retention with swelling ankles. The general conclusion is that the dangers outweigh the possible benefits.

For the Future

Ipriflavone, a preparation based on an organic extract from plants, promises a new, non-hormonal approach to the prevention and treatment of bone disease. So far, studies in Italy, Japan and Hungary have shown promising results with few reported side-effects (mainly gastro intestinal upsets and skin rashes). The research programme is continuing in the UK and it will take a couple of years before full results show if treatment is effective. But the prospects are exciting and could mean that women who cannot take HRT will be offered a viable alternative.

A compound containing essential fatty acids could be yet another new way to treat osteoporosis. Essential fatty acids are substances found in many foods but some scientists think we may not be getting enough of them and the new compound could stop calcium loss from bones.

OSTEO-RELIEF:

Bone-Booster exercises for those who suffer from osteoporosis

YOU'RE NEVER TOO OLD to improve bone and muscle strength, even if you actually suffer from osteoporosis. Before-and-after research with very elderly people has demonstrated the benefit of bone-loading exercise and also shown how mobility and muscle power enhance even simple activities like getting up from a chair, lifting parcels or going up stairs. Of course, these benefits also reduce the risk of falling and suffering a fracture. Should you have the bad luck to fall, you're less likely to suffer serious consequences.

One study showed that 30 exercising women with an average age of 84 showed bone gains of over 2% compared to an inactive group who lost over 3% of bone thickness when monitored by researchers for three years. What makes this study remarkable is that they did it sitting down! Their routine included knee lifts, toe taps, arm lifts, sideways bends, leg spreads. The exercisers worked out for 30 minutes a day, 3 days a week.

Thin old people are more likely to fracture their hips when they fall than their plumper contemporaries. Some researchers suspect that the fat acts as a kind of shock absorber. Hence the arrival of the energy-absorbent hip-protector, a padded device developed in Denmark that could be worn by anyone frail and elderly and at risk of damaging falls. At present it is being assessed, but one day a range of protectors may be available to buy or borrow.

An 8-week programme of 'high resistance' training followed by 10 elderly people in an American residential home resulted in spectacular gains in muscle strength. Muscles were more flexible afterwards too, another vital weapon in the fight against falling. Improvements in muscle strength can come within weeks of doing regular daily exercise, but bone-building takes longer. There may even be an initial period when bone gets slightly thinner, but after a year, improvement should be discernible.

If you already suffer from osteoporosis, there's no need for us to remind you of the discomfort and pain you experience.

If you have the disease in your spine, particularly in your lower-middle back below the ribs, you may be permanently bent over and unable to bear weight though your spine. In this case, we know, exercises are difficult and in some cases impossible to perform.

The best treatment for severe sufferers is pain-relieving drugs prescribed by the doctor and rest in bed with a pillow under the head for support. One pillow if possible, though we know some people can only find relief with more. Add a pillow under the knees and relax with legs straight if you find that more comfortable.

Most people, however, can benefit from some exercise, and we have designed our Osteo-Relief Bone Boosters specifically for osteoporosis sufferers. Do them on a regular basis for at least 3 months before you expect to see any improvement. Don't be discouraged if you feel initial discomfort. After a fall or operation, it is often difficult to overcome the pain barrier – the fear of pain, in fact. But remember the rewards in terms of regaining mobility, strength and independence, and try to stick it out.

If you have any doubts, show the exercises to your doctor or consult a trained physiotherapist. The extra stress on bones during exercise is not appropriate for people with advanced osteoporosis and could result in fracture. Seek medical advice if you think you are at risk before attempting Osteo-Relief Bone Boosters.

People without osteoporosis who have been actively exercising during their middle years can, and indeed do, continue at a high level of physical activity through out life, but late-starters need to take it nice and easy, putting the emphasis on walking, swimming, dancing and low-key routines like the one we suggest here.

A *brisk* daily walk is healthy and beneficial for anyone and everyone. Not only does it increase our stamina, strengthen our heart, improve circulation and tone up our muscles, but it's a Bone Booster too. A simple walk costs nothing and gives excellent results – so off your bottom and get those boots walking. Keep to a *brisk* pace and walk for at least 20 minutes. You should puff a bit!

THE PROGRAMME

The following 5 exercises are particularly beneficial if you already suffer from osteoporosis. They will help strengthen your spine and correct your posture.

1 Neck Retractions

Lie on your bed with your knees bent and a small pillow to support your head. Fix your eyes on a spot above you, and simply push with your neck and stick your chin up and out. Retract your chin and pull it down into your chest as far as you can. Continue with this 'chicken neck' exercise for 1 minute. As you progress over the weeks, remove the pillow but keep your knees bent and continue the exercise for 1 minute. Aim eventually to lie out on the floor without the pillow and with legs straight to do the exercise.

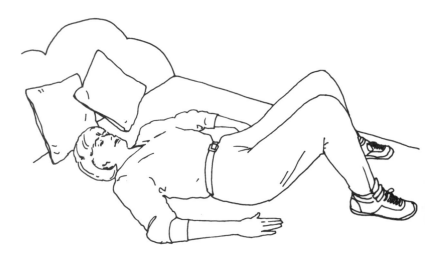

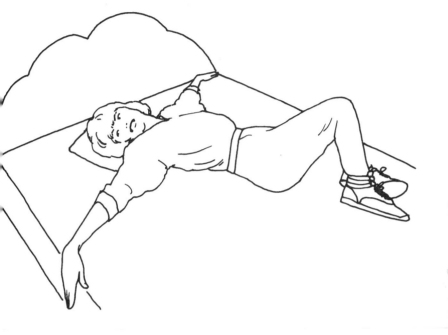

2 Spinal Rolls

Lie on your bed, preferably without a pillow, with both knees bent and arms out to your sides, palms down. Keep your feet in contact with the bed and roll both knees together over to your right side as far as comfortable. Try to look over to your left hand. Hold 2–4 seconds. Slowly bring your knees back to the centre, and carefully roll them over to your left side and try to look right. Hold 2–4 seconds. Keep your upper back, shoulders and arms in contact with the bed throughout the exercise. Aim to do 4 rolls to each side, and eventually to do the exercise on the floor.

3 Forward Lifts

To strengthen your tummy muscles lie on your bed with your head supported by a small pillow. Bend your knees up, feet down flat on the bed. Place your left hand behind your head (not neck), and extend your right hand on to your right thigh. Breathe out and lift your head and shoulders up, sliding your hand up to your knee. Breathe in and relax back down. Continue 4 times, then change hands and repeat 4 more lifts with your left hand on your left thigh. Aim eventually to do this exercise on the floor without a pillow, but always with your knees bent.

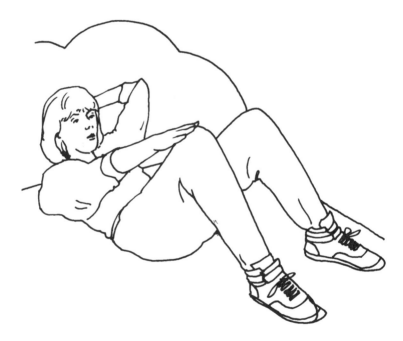

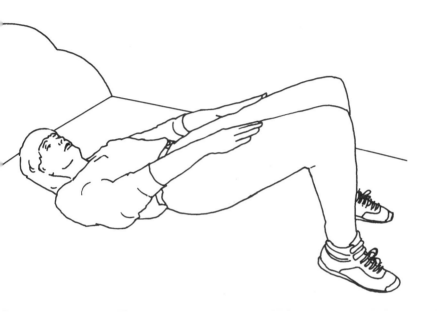

4 Bottom Lifts

Lie on your bed without a pillow, with your knees bent and feet flat down. Place your hands up on your thighs. Clench your bottom and lift it up off the bed. Hold for 2–4 seconds and carefully relax back down. Repeat 8 times, and try eventually to do this exercise on the floor.

5 Press Backs

This exercise is best performed on the floor. Lie out on your tummy, chin to floor. Place your hands under your shoulders with your fingers turned slightly inwards. Breathe out and push yourself back to lift your shoulders and chest up off the floor. Breathe in and relax back down. (Keep your chin facing down as you lift up.) Repeat this exercise 8 times.

When you first start this exercise you may need several pillows under your tummy in order to get comfortable and completely straight before attempting to bend backwards.

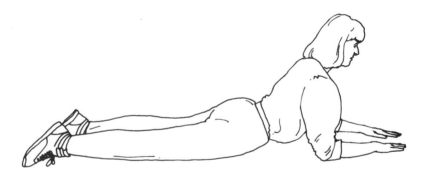

6 Relax

Lie on your back with your head supported by one pillow, (more may be necessary in severe cases). Place another pillow behind your knees and thighs to help relieve pain. Place your hands comfortably on your tummy. Breathe deeply, taking the breath into your abdomen, and feel the rise and fall of your tummy with your fingers. Close your eyes and relax.

It is often difficult for those who have vertebral fractures, with painful, tender spines and limited mobility, to lie on their backs. You may find it easier to try an alternative starting position for some of the exercises, such as sitting, from which you can do head and upper back exercises.

People who have already fractured their vertebrae can also benefit from exercise, to strengthen the muscles around the hips and knees – strong muscles in the legs help to prevent falls, which may well lead to fractures.

For information and further specific illustrated exercises for osteoporosis sufferers, contact the National Osteoporosis Society for their booklet Exercise and Physiotherapy in the Prevention and Treatment of Osteoporosis. Their address can be found on page 128.

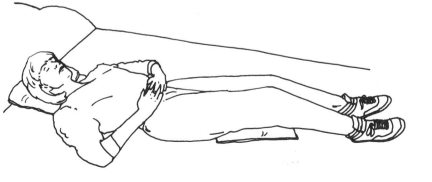

DAILY LIVING –
MAKING IT EASIER

Walk tall is tough advice if you suffer from a curved upper spine, but, nevertheless, it's exactly what you need. Get into the habit of checking that your shoulders are down and back, your chin pulled in and your weight evenly distributed. Hold your abdomen in if you can. Check your posture by standing against a wall: heels touching it, no hollow back. If you can't get your head straight against the wall at first, keep practising.

Don't slump when you sit, get your bottom well back into the chair. A soft, low armchair may seem like luxury, but if it makes you sink too low and rounds your back, change to something more upright with a high, firm back. A rolled towel at the back of your neck and another supporting the small of your back will enhance comfort and remind you to sit upright when reading. Make sure your feet are resting easily on the floor, and when you get up, resist bending forward. Keep as upright as possible and then stand up straight. You may find that at first you need to hold on to something as you get up, but gradually you'll be able to do it without the help.

A supporting mattress doesn't have to be iron-hard, and you don't need special orthopaedic types. On the other hand, it shouldn't sag. Buy a new one if yours shows signs of wear, and if it feels a bit on the hard side after that comforting sag, put a quilt over it and sleep on that to soften the blow.

Practise getting up and down from the floor once a day. It will help lessen the impact should you accidentally fall. Start by standing beside a steady, upright chair, holding the back with the left hand. Get down on your left knee, keeping your back straight, then take the right knee down, letting go of the chair and go down on all fours. Swing your bottom over to the floor on the right and sit down. Stand up in your own time, using the chair as support.

Guard your back when lifting anything heavy. Get as close to the object as possible, go down on one knee to pick it up, hug the load to your abdomen and lift with the strength from your legs by pushing down firmly with both feet. Don't try to take on too-heavy loads.

Remember, calcium helps reduce bone loss in older women. Recommended daily allowances are given on page 89 and calcium supplements have been shown to have a protective effect.

Poor diet not only leads to malnutrition and muscle weakness, it can also mean shrunken jaws and loose-fitting false teeth. Cooking for one doesn't have to be a chore. Even if someone else does the shopping for you, when it's cold and wintry outside, make sure you give them a shopping list that includes daily helpings of fresh fruit and vegetables, fish and dairy produce, and not too much fried food.

How to prevent falls

- Get rid of loose rugs, avoid slippery floors.
- Get better lighting, especially in hall and on stairs.
- Have a good grip handle on bath, and a non-slip mat in it.
- Get eyesight checked regularly.
- Keep a hall or landing light on at night.
- Watch out for uneven pavements – use a walking stick to help keep your balance.
- Wear well-fitting, supporting, non-slip shoes.

CONTACTS

Osteoporosis Dorset,
Dorset HealthCare, Trust
Headquarters, Shelley Road,
Bournemouth, Dorset BH1 4JQ.
Tel: (0202) 443064.

National Osteoporosis Society,
PO Box 10, Radstock, Bath,
Somerset BA3 3YV.
Tel: (0761) 432472.
Helpline, Tel: (0761) 431594.

Yoga for Health Foundation,
Ickwell Bury, Biggleswade,
Bedfordshire SG18 9EF.
Tel: (0767) 267271 (will supply list
of teachers offering remedial yoga
and standard yoga).

British Wheel of Yoga,
1 Hamilton Place, Boston Road,
Sleaford, Lincolnshire NG34 7ES
24-hour telephone no: (0529)
306851 (for local yoga teachers
throughout the country).

The Amarant Trust,
The Churchill Clinic, 80 Lambeth
Road, London SE1 7PW
Tel: (071) 401 3855 (for advice on
the menopause and HRT).

Women's Health Concern,
83 Earls Court Road,
London W8 6EF.
Tel: (071) 938 3932 (send Stamped
Addressed Envelope for information
regarding the menopause).

The Family Planning Clinic,
27/35 Mortimer Street,
London W1N 7RJ.
Tel: (071) 636 7866.

National Dairy Council,
5/7 John Princes Street,
London W1M 0AP.
Tel: (071) 499 7822 (for
information regarding calcium).

Well Women Clinics
NHS Menopausal Clinics
Contact your local hospital Bone
Screening Clinics

London Central YMCA,
Training and Development
Department, 12 Bedford Square,
London WC1B.
Tel: (071) 580 2989 (for
information regarding 50+ exercise-
to-music classes and teacher
training).

The Exercise Association of England
(formerly ASSET)
Unit 4, Angel Gate, City Road,
London EC1V 2PT (for information
on safe and effective exercise classes
throughout the country).

Extend,
1a North Street, Sheringham,
Norfolk NR26 8LJ.
Tel: (0158) 2832760 (exercise
training for older people and those
with disabilities of any age).

Women's Nutritional
Advisory Service,
PO Box 268, Lewes,
East Sussex, BN7 2QN.
Tel: (0273) 487366 (offers a
combined programme of non-
hormonal treatment, exercise and
nutrition).